# LIVING PLANTFULLY

## YOUR GUIDE TO GROWING, COOKING AND LIVING A HEALTHY, HAPPY & SUSTAINABLE PLANT-BASED LIFE

Lindsey Harrad

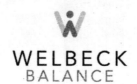

WELBECK
BALANCE

# ABOUT THE AUTHOR

Lindsey Harrad is an editor and writer with over 20 years' experience, including stints as lead feature writer and managing editor at *Vegetarian Living* magazine, the UK's best-selling and award-winning national vegetarian food and lifestyle title. She is currently completing her training to become a nutritional therapist.

Published in 2022 by Welbeck Balance
An imprint of Welbeck Non-Fiction Ltd
Part of Welbeck Publishing Group
Based in London and Sydney
www.welbeckpublishing.com

A CIP catalogue record for this book is available from the British Library.

ISBN
Hardback – 978-1-80129-025-8

Typeset by Steve Williams Creative
Printed in Great Britain by CPI Group (UK) Ltd, Croydon CR0 4YY

10 9 8 7 6 5 4 3 2 1

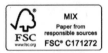

**Note/Disclaimer**
Welbeck Balance encourages diversity and different viewpoints.
However, all views, thoughts and opinions expressed in this book are the
author's own and are not necessarily representative of Welbeck Publishing Group as an
organization. All material in this book is set out in good faith for general guidance; Welbeck
Publishing Group makes no representations or warranties of any kind, express or implied, with
respect to the accuracy, completeness, suitability or currency of the contents of this book, and
specifically disclaims, to the extent permitted by law, any implied warranties of merchantability
or fitness for a particular purpose and any injury, illness, damage, death, liability or loss
incurred, directly or indirectly from the use or application of any of the information contained
in this book. This book is not intended to replace expert medical or psychiatric advice.
It is intended for informational purposes only and for your own personal use and guidance.
It is not intended to diagnose, treat or act as a substitute for professional medical advice.
The author and the publisher are not medical practitioners nor counsellors, and professional
advice should be sought before embarking on any health-related programme.

*For Maia and Alfie,*
*who are always in touch with their inner wild child.*
*I love you to the moon and back.*

# CONTENTS

# PART 3 — LIVE

# INTRODUCTION

"The relationship between people and nature
must be one of interdependence, otherwise
we risk overlooking something that indigenous
peoples have known all along: that we are nature
and nature is us, and failing to see this simple
truth is what has gotten us into this mess
in the first place."

**Tonio Sadik**, Senior Director, Environment, Lands and
Water, Assembly of First Nations (Canada)

**P**LANTS ARE POWERFUL – RADIANT WITH BEAUTY AND goodness, they represent the abundance that this generous and resilient Earth provides, and I'm on a mission to inspire everyone to get more of them onto our plates, and into our homes and gardens. Our health, and that of the planet, depends on it.

The philosophy of *Living Plantfully* is founded on the belief that we need a holistic, non-judgemental, label-free approach to phasing out animal products and focusing on plant alternatives in the kitchen and throughout the home. It's a journey that can be taken in a way that suits each individual or family, by making small changes at your own pace. And most importantly, it should be a joyful and life-enhancing experience too. This book not only explores the benefits of eating more plant-based foods, but also how to infuse every aspect of your life with the amazing properties of plants.

Like many people, I'm worried about climate change. I have young children, and I want their future on this planet to be safe and secure. But I didn't want to write a scary, pessimistic book about how the future might look if we can't prevent climate change, because I know that too much doom and gloom can lead to inaction. The world is facing up to some big issues and the scale of the problem often feels overwhelming and impossible for any one person to solve. But when we all make small changes, the collective effects can have a tremendous impact.

I decided we needed a book that would be informative but uplifting, inspiring and hopeful, filled with the promise of a positive way of living that celebrates deliciousness, kindness, health and happiness, while encouraging a form of "gentle activism" by choosing a lifestyle that shows love to our bodies, to our wider communities, to the other living creatures that share our world, and to the environment.

*Living Plantfully* can help you live your best life, while giving the planet its best chance for the future too.

# WHAT IS "LIVING PLANTFULLY"?

If I could distil the core message of this book down to one sentence, it would be this: everything that is naturally good for us, is good for the planet.

The philosopher Schopenhauer said, "health is not everything, but without health, everything is nothing." It's also true to say that we are nothing without a healthy planet to inhabit. Reducing our reliance on animal products and growing more plant foods – in the right place, in the right way – will not only improve our health, it will reduce greenhouse gas emissions and enrich the soil for growing a more exciting variety of crops. Rewilding our world by growing more trees and lavishing love on our gardens and green spaces supports biodiversity, reduces carbon levels and creates a more resilient food supply, as well as improving our physical and mental wellbeing.

"Living plantfully" is about so much more than food. While change often starts in the kitchen, becoming more interested in plant-centred health and wellbeing quite naturally goes hand-in-hand with an interest in more natural ways of cleaning, nature-based beauty and self-care, indoor and outdoor gardening, growing herbs and vegetables, foraging for wild foods and spending more time immersed in nature in the great outdoors. In a tech-heavy, stressful and increasingly urban modern world, we can all improve our quality of life by finding time for mindfulness – in whatever form most appeals to us – and making deeper connections with nature in our homes and beyond.

For most of the last decade, I was the editor of *Vegetarian Living* magazine; the best-selling vegetarian magazine in the UK, where I had the wonderful job of celebrating the best of meat-free cooking and providing ideas and inspiration for living a plant-centred, more sustainable life. I've had the privilege of meeting and talking to a great many interesting people, including chefs, restaurateurs, celebrities, gardeners, producers and other champions of food, wellness and green living. From these incredibly knowledgeable and passionate people, I've gained a broad view of how nutrition, health and sustainability interconnect in so many ways. It's been an enlightening journey, discovering a wide range of perspectives on the complex and fascinating issues that affect both people and the planet.

In *Living Plantfully*, I pull together all the wisdom and knowledge I've acquired and shape it into a holistic guide for a healthier, happier life, inviting you to make changes at your own pace and in a way that works for you. There's no pressure here, and no need to give yourself a label or define yourself by what you eat and how you choose to live. There are many people who don't connect with the idea of being labelled as a "vegetarian" or "vegan", but they do care deeply about where their food comes from. They want to improve their wellbeing and their chances of living a long and happy life by eating a healthier, more varied diet. They're interested in doing their bit to tackle climate change, and they're keen to make more ethical buying decisions to ensure both people and animals are treated with care and respect.

Living more "plantfully" can achieve all these things, and you don't have to categorize yourself to do it. Your hierarchy of personal values is yours alone to figure out – whether your priority is to buy organic for health reasons, to prioritize animal welfare by buying vegan products or to reduce your individual carbon footprint. There's no one ideal way to live or a perfect option in every situation; you just have to go with your gut and make what feels like the best choices for you.

When you give yourself permission to forget about labels and just start focusing on eating and living more mindfully, this can empower you to make healthier choices and form new habits at your own pace, with less pressure and no fear of "failure" or "cheating", or judgement from friends, family or an online community. You don't have to make any big announcements or clear your cupboards of "forbidden' foods", or take any drastic action at all – just start making some small, gradual changes.

This way of life is not about self-denial or following any set rules, it's simply about eating a greater abundance of vibrant, delicious plants and connecting with the power of nature in every aspect of your life.

# A HEALTHIER LIFE

Meat isn't entirely to blame for the current global health or climate crises, of course, but if people ate more beetroot than burgers the impact on both would be enormous. There is a well-established link between diet, wellbeing and life expectancy, and the growing availability of nutritionally depleted ultra-processed foods is a major contribution to the rapidly growing problem of obesity, mental health issues, diet-related diseases and premature death in wealthier nations.

Much of this poor health could be avoided with a deliciously simple prescription to eat more nourishing plant foods. Although most diet advice has tended to centre on the ideal balance of macronutrients – carbohydrates, fat and protein – for maintaining a healthy weight and preventing chronic diseases, the science is now telling us to be much more concerned about the micronutrients. It's those minute quantities of essential vitamins, minerals and phytonutrients that are so rich in plant foods, along with the "missing macronutrient" – fibre – that play such a nuanced role in our general wellbeing, from maintaining a healthy balance in our gut microbiome to reducing the damaging effects of inflammation in our bodies. Simply eating more minimally processed whole plant foods could transform human health on a global level, and it's far cheaper and simpler to eat more fruit and veg than it is to prop up the population's failing health with drugs and medical treatment.

Giving up or reducing meat and animal products is not automatically going to improve your health, of course. Whether you choose to be plant-based (adopting a diet exclusively or predominantly consisting of plant foods) or vegan (completely excluding all animal products in both diet and all areas of life) or something "flexitarian" in-between, there are still plenty of opportunities to eat ultra-processed foods or too many refined carbohydrates and sugary foods, as crisps, sweets, chocolate and wine can all be vegan too. It's also true that balanced diets containing moderate amounts of good-quality meat, fish and dairy can still be healthy.

5

However, the scientific evidence in favour of a plant-centred lifestyle is compelling. For a better chance of good health and a long life, a diet packed with an abundance of vegetables, fruits, beans, pulses, wholegrains, nuts and seeds is the best medicine. The good news is that you don't have to feel deprived, because when you take some or all of the meat, eggs and dairy off your plate, you make space for more vibrant, varied and flavoursome foods.

## A WEALTHIER LIFE

There's a widespread belief that eating plant-based foods is more expensive and therefore inaccessible to people on lower incomes, although often this misconception is based on people buying readymade products or fashionable exotic ingredients when they go vegan. Regardless, food bills continue to spiral upward, supermarkets rarely run promotions on fresh produce – while the cheapest deals are for the most nutritionally empty processed products – and a combination of busy lifestyles and endless temptation from convenience foods make it harder to eat well.

However, you can choose how and where to spend your budget to make it go further, making good food and better health a priority for you and your family. Techniques such as batch cooking homemade dishes for your freezer for a fraction of the cost of readymeals makes good sense for everyone, on any budget. If you can spend a bit of time and energy reinventing your recipe repertoire and learning new skills, you'll naturally find more pleasure in cooking from scratch, and hopefully get excited about trying new ingredients too. Cooking more mindfully also means reducing food waste, which saves you money and helps to reduce global warming.

Finally, there's the simple fact that most plant protein is cheaper than meat. A bag of lentils or chickpeas (garbanzo beans) costs far less than a pack of chicken and again, if you cook from scratch, the food always goes further. If you build on savings by living plantfully in other ways, such as making natural cleaning products and growing your own herbs or vegetables, even in a small way, you'll start to cut costs even more. Living a simpler, more natural, pared-back life saves money, but also brings so many other rewards.

Cooking beautiful food for friends and family is an expression of love, and it can be a form of self-love – or self-care – too; consider it an investment in your health and wellbeing.

## A MORE SUSTAINABLE LIFE

While the most compelling personal motivation for change is the potential to live a longer, happier, healthier life, as an attractive side benefit it could also be a big part of the solution for the climate change crisis.

The latest figures suggest that food production contributes 35% of all manmade greenhouse gas emissions, with meat and dairy causing twice as many emissions as plant foods.[1] This means that how we shop for, cook, eat and dispose of food is now recognized to be the single most important factor in our personal eco footprint. It doesn't mean you have to be completely vegan, but even making small changes to individual eating habits can have a substantial collective impact on preserving the planet's resources and slowing the pace of climate change. Look at other sustainability initiatives that have been successful, such as encouraging people to switch to reusable water bottles or to turn the central heating down by 1 degree. They are super simple to do, and they also save us money. It's a win-win situation. Research suggests that if we all switched to a predominantly plant-based diet, greenhouse gas emissions could be reduced by as much as 52%.[2] Research analysis by Oxford University scientist Joseph Poore shows that if every family in the UK alone swapped a red meat meal to a plant-based meal just once a week, the environmental impact would be the same as taking 16 million cars off the road. Which is not a bad start. Imagine what we could achieve if four, five or six meals a week were veggie or vegan?

Despite the growing vegan trend, the global appetite for animal products is worryingly insatiable – while the population has doubled in size, consumption of animal products has quadrupled since the 1960s. The Food and Agriculture Organisation of the United Nations predicts that by 2050 world meat production will have almost doubled again, as demand for meat, eggs and dairy products continues to grow.[3]

If you already have concerns about animal welfare, then you probably know that it's simply not possible to produce meat, fish, dairy and eggs on this scale in a humane way, without commoditizing and exploiting livestock in large-scale intensive farming systems. There's also the fact that livestock need to eat too. The world's cattle alone consume a quantity of food equal to the calorific needs of 8.7 billion people – more than the entire human population on Earth. The vast swathes of land used to graze animals and grow feed could be far better used for growing crops for direct human consumption, reducing greenhouse gas emissions, deforestation and the loss of even more biodiversity.

The consensus among scientists working on environmental issues is that we need a radical global shift toward plant-based eating to help reverse climate change. This is not a fad diet; plants are the food of the future.

## A HAPPIER LIFE

Engagement with nature has a particularly potent influence on our mental and physical wellbeing, and simple activities such as growing flowers or vegetables, walking in nature, exercising outdoors and even filling our homes and workspaces with houseplants have all been shown to have scientifically measurable effects on health and happiness.

Plant powers go well beyond those we ingest; they make our world habitable, with trees purifying the air we breathe, sequestering carbon and enriching the atmosphere with oxygen in return, even emitting soothing chemicals that have been shown to lower blood pressure. Just being surrounded by the green, leafy loveliness of plants – both indoors and out – exerts a calming, positive influence.

Gardening, too, has extraordinary healing powers, boosting wellness in countless ways, from producing deliciously nourishing things to eat, to exposing us to the beneficial bacteria in the soil and building a sense of community. The more plants we grow, the more we promote local biodiversity and support healthy ecosystems, while also enjoying the visual and edible delights of a vibrant and productive garden.

Making a deeper connection with nature will enrich your life and strengthen your resolve to live in a kinder, more plant-centred way. Every small step you can take, from showing compassion for animals and the environment by reducing your meat intake, to growing some vegetables or spending more time in nature, is a positive move toward living in a way that benefits people, planet and animals, and your own health and wellbeing.

We all need a bit more awe of nature in our lives – and we don't have to travel to exotic far-flung destinations to find it. It's everywhere we look, and everyone can enjoy the incredible bounty that nature provides. Step outside, it's all yours.

## RECIPES

Scattered throughout the following chapters are some simple recipes and suggestions, and I've also provided a list of useful books and other sources of plant-based inspiration in the resources section at the back of this book. You can find more delicious recipes online by visiting my website www.livingplantfully.co.uk

# HOW TO USE THIS BOOK

Divided into three sections – Grow, Cook and Live – each chapter explores a different aspect of living a plant-centred life, opening with a no-pressure goal and providing inspiration for putting plants at the heart and centre of the way you live and eat.

I have opened with Grow, as I believe gardening is the most inclusive of all the plant-based ideas and activities suggested in this book. Anyone can take pleasure in growing, whether that's a single pot of herbs on a windowsill or joining a community tree-planting project. Growing on any scale is a wonderful way to develop a deeper appreciation for plants and the health benefits they bring as we tend them in the garden and cook with them in the kitchen.

Plants nourish our mental and physical health in so many ways from plot to plate, and the Cook section explores some of the delicious ways we can include more of them in our diet.

Finally, in Live, we discover how to live more plantfully in the home, from self-care and cleaning inspired by nature to the pleasures of nurturing house plants.

At the end of each chapter, I've provided signposts to other relevant sections that relate to the issues and ideas mentioned as, inevitably, many are interlinked. This book is designed to be read chronologically, but each chapter is self-contained, too, so it's also ideal for dipping into when you need advice and inspiration on a particular topic.

# 1

# LET'S ALL BE TREE HUGGERS

"In nature, nothing is perfect and everything is perfect."

Alice Walker

**E**VERY SIGN OF NATURE AT WORK IS A PRECIOUS GIFT.
In winter, on a walk along mud-slicked footpaths, the sight of the first pensive heads of snowdrops peeping through the earth is a watershed moment: spring is stirring underground. Like generations before us, we measure our days by seasonal signs, from blossom buds appearing on boughs above, to swathes of cheery daffodils followed by wood-dwelling bluebells, and later apples clustered in autumnal orchards.

Not all of nature's work is showy, and we can still find pleasure in her smallest intricate details and sensory pleasures – from the textures of craggy crevices on ancient tree trunks, to the colours of delicate fronds of living lichens on rocks, walls, twigs and bark; or the aroma of wild garlic lingering in the woods.

We all need to reconnect with our inner wildness. Humankind's existence is only a tiny dot on Earth's vast timeline, and although the proportion of time in which we've started separating ourselves from the natural environment through building and industrialization is also relatively tiny and has happened over just a few generations, in terms of evolution – which moves at a much slower pace than advances in technology – we haven't had time to adapt as a species. This could be one of the reasons we are seeing so many people experiencing mental and physical health problems. For humans – who are as much part of nature as any other living creature – living in a suffocating world of steel and concrete is not our natural state of being.

This book, will explore the myriad ways that a holistic, plant-focused life can enhance your quality of life. While eating more whole plant foods is an important lifestyle change that has almost instant benefits to our wellbeing, the other side of the health equation is exercise, and we now know that a healthy lifestyle should also include some outdoor activity in nature.

Walking anywhere improves blood flow, makes your heart pump more efficiently, helps to maintain bone density and joint health, balances blood sugar levels, boosts energy and tops up your Vitamin D stores, and just half an hour of brisk walking is enough to make a positive impact on your health. It's now believed to be even more beneficial than a gym session, as research shows that walking in nature reduces blood pressure more than walking on a treadmill or in a busy urban area.

The importance of incidental activity for good health, and specifically longevity, is supported by studies of "Blue Zones", which first evolved out of research conducted by Gianni Pes and Michel Poulain in Sardinia, where there were an unusually high number of male centenarians (people living beyond 100). One factor people living in Blue Zones – which include places such as Ikaria, Greece and Okinawa, Japan – have in common is that they all walk a lot. While not necessarily doing much, or any, formal exercise, their levels of "natural movement" are high thanks to their often traditional lifestyles (including growing their own vegetables and having no mod cons to do household jobs), and they also have diets low in meat and high in plant foods, beans and pulses in particular. There were other beneficial factors, such as low levels of stress, being in a loving relationship, having a close extended family nearby and having a sense of purpose in their lives, and while this research was not a controlled scientific study,  there's no doubt we can learn a thing or two about diet and exercise from these savvy centenarians who are active in ways that human beings have evolved naturally to be. In this way, we too can live longer and healthier lives.

The problem is that many of us are not doing enough of any kind of activity – globally, 1 in 4 adults don't exercise enough based on the World Health Organization's recommendation of a minimum of 150 minutes a week – and modern life with its screens and sofa-based entertainments means we aren't doing a lot of incidental activity in our work or leisure time. With adults in the UK and US averaging 9–10 hours a day of sitting, encouraging everyone to build a daily walk into their routine could go a long way toward improving overall physical and mental wellness and life expectancy.

"Sitting is the new smoking" has become an oft-quoted slogan to put the fear of sloth into us. It's true that sitting for long periods of time is thought to slow our metabolism, which affects the body's ability to regulate blood sugar and blood pressure, and break down body fat, even if we do a workout every day. Regular, frequent interruptions such as standing up or walking around for a few minutes can help by switching on your muscles and your metabolism just enough to reduce levels of blood sugar and fat and counteract other negative effects of being sedentary. But don't get overly anxious if you do have a sedentary job – it's all about balance. Studies show that leisure-time sitting has a stronger link with poor health than sitting for work, so just make sure that when you're not working, you're being active – especially if your job means spending long hours sitting at a desk – whether that's formal exercise, an outdoor walk, or just keeping busy around the house and garden.

The simplest way to combine the amazing benefits of exercise and being in nature is to be active in an outdoor space. This could be a walk, doing some gardening or moving your workout or yoga session to your local park. The wonderful thing about exercising outdoors is that anyone can do it and it requires no expensive equipment or monthly membership fee.

# FIVE REASONS TO GO FOR A WALK IN THE WILD

It might feel counter-intuitive to go for a walk when you're feeling tired, lacking in energy or in a low mood, but it's often the best thing you can do to make yourself feel better. If you need more motivation, here are five evidence-backed reasons for finding time for a daily walk. If you can't readily access a green space or countryside in the time you have available – a brisk walk anywhere still has many health benefits.

## 1 TO MAKE YOU FEEL HAPPIER

Walking generates a feel-good effect. It's so powerful that walking not only improves self-esteem, relieves anxiety and reduces stress, it can cut your risk of becoming depressed by 30%.[1] Walking boosts your mood by increasing blood flow and circulation throughout your body and brain, which has a positive effect on your central nervous system, or your hypothalamic-pituitary-adrenal (HPA) axis, which regulates your stress response. As you walk, you are actively calming your nerves and reducing your stress levels, which in turn has many positive benefits for wellbeing, beyond just making you feel happier.

## 2 TO GET A HEALTHY DOSE OF MICROBES

It's not just gardening that exposes us to beneficial bacteria (see chapter 3 for more on this), research suggests that going for a walk outside in a green space – including urban locations such as city parks – increases the diversity of bacteria found in the nose and on the skin.[2] This microbial transfer from the environment may have a beneficial impact on your microbiome and support both your gut health and immunity.

## 3 TO SLEEP BETTER

Being outside in natural light helps to regulate our sleep patterns. When the sun sets, it helps our brains to release the right levels of melatonin to get a good-quality sleep. Walking first thing in the morning is particularly beneficial as exposure to daylight soon after you wake up reduces your melatonin production first thing, helping you feel wide awake and setting you up for a more productive day.

## 4 TO BOOST YOUR IMMUNE SYSTEM AND REDUCE INFLAMMATION

A regular dose of just 20 minutes of physical activity such as brisk walking has been shown to stimulate the immune system and produce an anti-inflammatory response at cellular level. When your brain and sympathetic nervous system are activated by exercise (including accelerated heart rate and raised blood pressure), hormones are released into the blood stream, in turn triggering an immunological response. This includes the production of many cytokines (proteins) including TNF, which is an important regulator of inflammation, and which also helps boost immune responses.[3] Although inflammation is part of your body's natural defence system and is designed to defend against attack from viruses and other invaders, chronic inflammation can be very damaging to health and is associated with several serious conditions such as type-2 diabetes – so this is a great reason to get your trainers on.

## 5 TO DEVELOP YOUR NEXT BIG IDEA

Many of the great philosophers, from Aristotle to Kierkegaard, believed that they did their best thinking while walking. With each step, blood flow to the brain increases, and this helps improve your memory, cognitive function and can prevent against decline as you age. The positive sensory stimulation of walking in nature can release those creative juices, too, and experts suggest that if you can find time to walk in the morning, perhaps before work, you can also boost your energy and mental clarity for the whole day. As the philosopher Nietzsche once wrote, "All truly great thoughts are conceived by walking."

# THE NATURE CURE

There's a particularly powerful synergy between walking and being in nature that operates on a physical, mental and even spiritual level. Connecting with nature is hugely important for mental wellbeing. At a time when the UK charity Mind reports that 1 in 4 people every year will experience a mental health issue, one simple and low-cost way of managing these conditions, or even just enhancing our general sense of wellbeing, is to top up our nature exposure.

You may have heard of "nature deficit disorder", which, while not being an officially recognized psychological condition, is a concept that has gained traction since writer Richard Louv coined the term in his book, *Last Child in the Woods*. Louv's argument was that we are all spending more time indoors, especially children, and that this makes us feel alienated from nature or more likely to suffer from problems such as low moods or poor concentration.

Spending just a few hours every week outdoors in green spaces is the way to redress the balance. A recent study of 20,000 people, led by researchers from the University of Exeter, discovered that two hours a week spent in nature is the benchmark for enjoying the benefits of better health and psychological wellbeing.[4] These benefits applied to all participants, regardless of age, gender and socio-economic background, and even those with disabilities or pre-existing health conditions. Crucially, these 120 minutes can be spread across several shorter outings and applied to any nature-rich settings, such as town parks, the beach or woodlands, proving you don't have to do long treks in the wilderness to reap the rewards.

The idea that spending time in nature can create a happier society has even been quantified financially in a recent study from the UK's Forest Research, which reports that walks in UK woodlands save the National Health Service £185 million a year in mental health treatment costs, while street trees cut a further £16 million a year from the NHS antidepressant bill.[5]

One way to further top up your happiness levels is to take weekly "awe walks", where you make a conscious effort to shift your focus outward instead of inward, soaking up the sights, sounds and even smells of nature you experience on the way. You know that feeling when you stand at the top of a mountain and feel as though the whole world is at your feet, or find yourself alone on a beach in winter and experience the exhilaration of the waves crashing onto the shore? Coming face to face with nature's power and magnificence is the moment we understand our place in the universe and it helps us learn to look beyond ourselves and our own daily worries. Scientists have discovered that experiencing a sense of awe in nature – that awareness of something larger than the self – leads to feeling more optimistic and coping better with stress, as well as boosting positive emotions such as gratitude and compassion.[6] Researchers conducting the study in California even reported that, for the people participating, the smiles on their selfies were bigger after taking an awe walk, even if taking just one 15-minute walk a week.

If you fancy trying it, plan a regular outing to somewhere that inspires awe – it doesn't have to be Niagara Falls to have an effect, it could just be a glorious view of the countryside from a high vantage point, or experiencing a spectacular sunset. Use your awe walk as an opportunity to make new discoveries. The point is to switch off the buzzing in your brain and bring a sense of pure childlike wonder to your appreciation of nature. When you stop and really soak in every detail of your surroundings, you can't help but see, feel and hear just how awesome nature really is – and it does help to put your own problems into perspective.

## MINDFUL MOMENTS

While brisk walking is beneficial for physical and mental health, it's also good to slow down the pace sometimes, and introduce a deeper element of mindfulness to your time spent outdoors, appreciating the smallest details of nature's creation, as well as the bigger "wow" moments. You've probably heard of "forest bathing" or *shinrin-yoku*, a physiological and psychological exercise that originated in Japan in the 1980s as a natural antidote to over-exposure to urban environments and technology, and also to inspire people to reconnect with and protect the country's forests. But how is "forest bathing" any different to just taking a walk in the woods?

"It's completely different," says Sonya Dibbin, a forest bathing practitioner and founder of Adore Your Outdoors in Hampshire. "Forest bathing is all about deepening your connection with nature by moving slowly, being peaceful, pressing pause and engaging your senses. There's a lot of stillness involved – I often recommend people lie on the forest floor during our sessions."

The most important difference between a walk and forest bathing is that it's not exercise, it's a mindfulness practice. During forest bathing, you don't travel very far, there's no goal of hitting 10,000 steps or raising your heart rate into the cardio zone, everything is very, very slow. Silence, stillness and no distracting chit-chat are important for really engaging with the forest surroundings.

"People find it amazing that they can spend ten minutes looking at a hazel leaf and they get very absorbed in noticing the veins, the textures, the colours," says Sonya. "All this detail goes unnoticed on a conventional brisk walk where exercise is the goal. Our forest bathing sessions run for three hours because the scientific evidence shows that to be physiologically beneficial – in other words, to induce a reduction in the production of cortisol, the stress hormone – we must spend at least two hours mindfully immersed in nature."

As for tree hugging, Sonya says it does sometimes happen on her courses. "I just think that we've got into a right old pickle as a society when hugging a tree is seen as something laughable and you'd be ridiculed for it, but it's seen as perfectly fine to spend 95% of our lives indoors connected to technology, doing things that aren't healthy for us," she says. "It's crazy really. But I do think we've turned a corner, attitudes are definitely changing."

## A BREATH OF FRESH AIR

As anyone who enjoys a stroll in the woods will know, there's nothing like taking a deep breath of air among the trees; it has a distinctive aroma of earthy hummus from the soil and a clean freshness that is unique to woodland. "Forest air is the epitome of healthy air," says Peter Wohlleben, in his fascinating book *The Hidden Life of Trees*. "People who want to take a deep breath of fresh air or engage in physical activity in a particularly agreeable atmosphere step out into the forest.

... The air truly is considerably cleaner under the trees, because the trees act as huge air filters."

If we didn't already know that trees are incredibly beneficial for our health, they also filter particles of pollutants, such as soot, dust, acids, toxic hydrocarbons and nitrogen compounds from the air and keep them trapped in their canopy, well away from our lungs. Trees also release oxygen when water and the carbon dioxide they breathe in are broken down during photosynthesis and, particularly during the daytime in the summer months, they can release around 29 tons of oxygen per square mile of woodland. We breathe in nearly two pounds of oxygen every 24 hours, which is why a walk in the woods literally feels like a breath of fresh air. But trees – especially conifers – also emit phytoncides, which are defensive chemicals that fight off harmful pests that might damage the tree. Phytoncides have antibiotic properties, and these chemicals create that unique, heady, forest scent – an aroma that becomes especially powerful on hot summer days.

In an intriguing example of how natural defensive compounds produced by plants can benefit human health, research suggests that we may benefit physiologically from inhaling phytoncides. "As we breathe in the phytoncides they are proven to lower our heart rate and reduce heart rate variability, so they bring a sense of calm," says Sonya. "They also increase the number and activity of white blood cells that help us fight off everything from cancer to viruses. You are genuinely boosting your immune system by breathing in the forest air."

Research has shown, though, that when you are walking through the woods at a fast pace with your heart pumping, you don't get the full benefits. These come from being slow, from inhaling and exhaling deeply and consciously, mindfully connecting with the forest. You enjoy these benefits when you leave the forest, too, as your stress levels remain lower for days afterwards.

So, on busy days, remind yourself that it's not self-indulgent to carve out a little time for connecting with the wild world. The more time you spend in nature, the more you appreciate the beautiful balance and synergy of this Earth and the importance of nurturing it, and it will also do your own wellbeing a power of good.

# MiNDFUL MANDALA-MAKiNG

Sonya suggests a natural gratitude exercise, which involves creating a mandala using found materials, and this is something you could do in the forest or at home in your garden. "I recommend thinking of something that you're feeling grateful for. It might be the place you're in, the weather or someone wonderful in your life. Then use natural materials to build them a gift," she says.

Mandalas can be incredibly intricate artworks, but your mandala could be a simple and beautiful arrangement of stones, shells, leaves, pinecones, twigs, driftwood or anything you find in abundance around you. Just start the piece even if you don't know what it will end up being – you will find your creativity flows and the mandala will emerge naturally.

When you've finished your design, allow yourself some time to reflect on your experience, and take a photo to capture your creation. Significantly, you will leave it in place for others to enjoy or the natural world to relocate or redesign. "There are a couple of important lessons involved; it's not just the finished result – the journey is also important, and acceptance that the things we put in place in our lives may not last forever. And that's okay," says Sonya.

## TEN WAYS TO INSPIRE YOUR DAILY WALKING PRACTICE

There's always an excuse not to go out for a walk – it's raining, you've got a report to write, the kitchen needs cleaning. If you're not in the habit of going for daily walks, knowing all the reasons you *should* is not nearly as motivating as going out because you *want* to. If you can find that reason to go that makes your heart sing, soon you'll move heaven and earth to make time for your daily walks.

## 1 MARKING THE SEASONS

The predictability of the seasons can be comforting, especially during difficult times, so make a point of marking seasonal events by, for example, going to find the first bluebells or rediscovering the joy of conker collecting. Recording your sightings and photographs in a journal or on social media helps you stay in touch with the seasonal cycles, and you can enjoy your nature diary even when you don't have time to go out for a walk.

## 2 REDISCOVERING CHILDHOOD PLEASURES

Do things the six-year-old you loved to do. Walk barefoot in the grass, crunch through autumn leaves, play Poohsticks, paddle in a stream, learn to identify wildflowers and draw your finds or, yes, hug a tree.

## 3 COMMUNITY SPIRIT

Get a friend or family member to come along. Join a walking group, take up an outdoor walking-based activity, such as golf or Nordic walking, group hikes or power walking, all of which will improve your social life, be a good form of exercise and provide a healthy dose of "Vitamin G" (G stands for green).

## 4 DISCOVER YOUR PASSION

Not everyone enjoys a walk just for a walk's sake. Finding a purpose for the walks can help. A daily walk to a quiet spot for sketching or writing a journal can unleash your creative potential.

## 5 GET THE FAMILY INVOLVED

Dog walking (you can "borrow" a dog through organizations that match busy owners with dog lovers, or volunteer to walk dogs at rescue centres if you don't have your own) or engaging activities such as geocaching can make family walks in nature more appealing, especially to older children.

## 6 FACTOR IN TIME TO PLAY

Simple additions to a family walk, such as taking along a fishing net for pond dipping or sketchbooks for bark rubbing, playing Eye Spy, or collecting leaves for scrapbooking or crafts, can make it feel more purposeful. Buying a field guide and learning to identify tree species or bird calls as a family is so satisfying and something children will never forget as they grow up.

## 7 FORAGING AND FEASTING

As the seasons change, go looking for wild foods, such as blackberries or apples; there's such joy in the hunt. Find foraging inspiration in chapter 12.

## 8 SIT QUIETLY

On your walks, take time to sit peacefully and enjoy a mindful moment. Tune into the sounds and sights around you, from the trills and chirps of birdsong to raindrops glistening on a spider's web or a squirrel darting about among the trees. Breathe deeply, inhale those phytoncides and release any anxiety and stress.

## 9 MAKE A WALK YOUR TEA BREAK

When you're ready to take a break from work, take your tea or coffee in a flask or travel cup and walk to your closest green space, even if it's just a park bench. Drink your tea outdoors, soak up the fresh air and head back to your desk feeling invigorated. Even 10 minutes each way is a 20-minute walk that you've squeezed into the day.

## 10 WINDOW WATCHING

When a walk really isn't possible, set aside 10 minutes to gaze out of the window or step into an outdoor space. Let the sound of the wind rustling in the trees provide a moment of calm and clarity. If you don't have a view of nature, look up – the sight of clouds scudding across the sky is so soothing. The predominant colour of nature – green – has been shown to be good for wellbeing, so if you really can't get away from your desk, spend some time tending to your houseplants or find a forest video online, as even looking at greenery on a screen has been shown to have some benefits.

# THE POWER OF FRACTALS

Fractals are repeated patterns that may appear to be chaotic but have order. They are found everywhere in nature, from leaves to fern fronds, pinecones and flowers, and even whole trees are fractals.

Research has shown that people enter a more relaxed state in nature because the fractal structure of our eyes often matches the fractal structures of the images we are looking at and this triggers a physiological stress-reducing response. This is why it's so relaxing to study trees and plants – and it can even work when looking at photographs of them.

# SIGNPOSTS

For more on:

🌱 Inflammation, *see* chapter 2

🌱 Health benefits of gardening, *see* chapter 3

🌱 Foraging ideas, *see* chapter 12

🌱 Why trees are good for us and the planet, *see* chapter 6

# 2

# PLANT SUPERSTARS

"It's so easy to lose that connection with food if we're not careful, and to forget we're cooking something that came from the earth. It's a very primal, natural thing and food today can spiral a long way from that."

Anna Jones, author, food writer
and *Observer* columnist

**T**AKE A TOMATO. EVERY SINGLE RED, PLUMP PACKAGE CONTAINS powerful, multi-tasking nutrients essential for sustaining life, which also help us look more radiant, feel energized and age gracefully. There's so much going on under the skin of fruit, vegetables and other plant foods that scientists are still making new discoveries about their health-boosting potential. They've only scratched the surface of understanding exactly how the nutrients in plants work individually and collectively to keep our bodies functioning at their best and prevent some of the leading lifestyle diseases that lead to poor health and lower life expectancy.

The word "collectively" is important. While a tomato may have remarkable powers, we wouldn't thrive on a diet of tomatoes alone. But we do have a rather reductionist way of thinking about food sometimes. For example, we might know that oats are a good source of soluble fibre, or that oranges provide vitamin C, and in this way, foods get put into little boxes that don't really do justice to the full range of their superpowers. Reducing any vegetable down to a single star quality is underselling it, because each is a complex package of essential vitamins, minerals and polyphenols wrapped up in fibre with a dazzling array of benefits for health. This is why all plants are superfoods. Not just the obscure ones with well-funded PR campaigns. You don't have to eat fashionable, expensive ingredients like kelp, dragon fruit or baobab (unless you want to) because affordable, everyday apples, broccoli and onions have amazing powers too.

No one ingredient is the only star; we must focus on the whole constellation and how they all work together to create a super-charged, nutrition-packed galaxy of goodness. Dr Rupy Aujla, creator of The Doctor's Kitchen, is an NHS doctor who has done brilliant work in the UK on making healthy, functional food more accessible (and delicious) through his podcast and books, expresses it perfectly: "We shouldn't be focusing specifically on including one particular vegetable or 'superfood', it's about the cumulative effect of all these healthy ingredients that you consume over weeks, months and years that have protective value when it comes to health conditions, and this is borne out by the science."[1]

# WHERE DO PLANT POWERS COME FROM?

Maybe you, like me, have often wondered why by some magical happenstance plants produce thousands of compounds that potentially reduce our chances of developing some of the most serious lifestyle diseases affecting millions of people across the globe each year? After all, these are not conditions that affect plants, so why do they hold the key to a cure, or at the very least, a chance of prevention? The simple answer is that they don't do it for us, of course. Plants mainly produce polyphenols for their own self-preservation, including defending themselves against environmental threats, such as ultraviolet radiation or attack from diseases or pests.[2] However, it's a stroke of serendipity for us.

Polyphenols are a group of beneficial compounds primarily found in fruit, vegetables, herbs, spices, coffee, tea, chocolate and red wine. Terms such as "polyphenols", "antioxidants" and "phytonutrients" are often used interchangeably and it can be confusing, so to clarify: the term "phytonutrients" is a broad name for the thousands of compounds produced by plants. One group of these compounds is called polyphenols, many of which can act as antioxidants, which means they can neutralize harmful free radicals that damage cells and cause inflammation. Polyphenols and other phytonutrients have been linked to so many processes in the body, with a staggering array of benefits from improved immunity to regulating blood sugar levels, reducing the incidence of breast and bowel cancer, blood clots, arthritis, osteoporosis, high blood pressure, depression, dementia – and even assisting with weight loss.

"Eating the rainbow" has become a key health message because it's a simple way to remember to eat whole fruit and vegetables of every hue, including the skins and leaves, which means you'll naturally get a diverse range of vitamins, minerals and phytonutrients and reap all the health rewards. The bright or dark colours and strong flavours of foods sometimes signal the presence of different health-enhancing polyphenols, such as the characteristic tannins and bitter flavours of green tea and coffee, or the purple hue of some berries and grapes, which get their colour from a flavonoid polyphenol called anthocyanin.

The contribution of phytonutrients to human health is complex and research is ongoing, but maybe all the average person looking to eat a more nourishing diet promoting health and longevity needs to know is that if a magic elixir exists that could help you live well for longer – phytonutrient-rich plant foods are it. And the good news is, the list of those foods includes red wine and dark chocolate – in moderation, of course.

## WHAT'S THE FUSS ABOUT INFLAMMATION?

Antioxidants have become a particularly hot topic in nutrition lately thanks to their important role in reducing inflammation. The best way to explain inflammation is to imagine you've cut your finger – the area immediately goes red and sore on the surface. Meanwhile, inside your body, proteins are released in response to the damage to your skin and these send signals to your immune system to prevent infection and heal the affected area. Without this rapid-response service, we'd be highly susceptible to bacterial infections that could lead to severe illness or even death. So, inflammation is certainly not a bad thing, it's a lifesaver.

However, inflammation is designed to be a relatively short and efficient response to trauma or infection, lasting only days or maybe weeks for a serious injury. However, thanks to a number of lifestyle factors, people are now experiencing low-grade inflammation – often called "meta-inflammation" – which is like a fire that keeps smouldering and never fully goes out. Over time, it's no less harmful because our bodies are not designed to be in a permanent state of inflammation and it can cause a range of symptoms from fatigue to not being able to focus, mood swings and at the more serious end of the scale, depression, high blood pressure, type-2 diabetes and heart disease.

The good news is that there's a cure for inflammation that's relatively inexpensive, accessible, with no adverse side effects and it's easy to start taking today – all you need is a prescription for eating more plant foods. What we eat is a key trigger for inflammation, and research shows that a predominantly plant-based, high-fibre diet, which includes healthy fats from plants such as nuts and seeds, and a low intake of animal protein and processed foods, is the simplest way to stop inflammation – and maintain a healthy weight. It's even more effective if it works in tandem with lifestyle changes such as eating slowly, reducing stress, taking up mindful activities such as yoga or meditation, walking every day (ideally in a natural environment), enjoying regular exercise and getting a good night's sleep. Even being more sociable and joining in with community activities has been shown to be beneficial. A holistic approach is the best way to dampen the smouldering embers of chronic inflammation.

# FUELLING PEOPLE AND PROTECTING THE PLANET

What we eat has such an enormous impact on every aspect of life on this Earth, from chemical reactions taking place at molecular level in the cells of our bodies when we ingest the nutrients from food, to farming practices that are fuelling global warming through activities such as deforestation. When it comes to climate change, one of the most significant environmental pollution concerns is greenhouse gases, of course, around a third of which come from agriculture.

While there's a huge and very lucrative industry dedicated to telling us what we should eat to achieve better health, a longer life and faster weight loss, the EAT-*Lancet* Commission's Planetary Health Diet is unique because it's the first to set universal scientific targets for a food system designed to keep both people and planet healthy.[3] A group of 37 scientists from around the world were tasked with the challenge of answering a simple question: "Can we feed a global population of 10 billion people a healthy diet within planetary boundaries?" Exploring every issue from farm to fork, the plan they presented is adaptable to anyone, living anywhere, whether they choose to eat meat and dairy or not. It recognizes that feeding the global population the most nutritious diet possible and slowing down the degradation of the planet are intrinsically linked, and that every nation needs to get on board and make radical changes to the way we grow and consume food to have any hope of meeting the UN Sustainable Development Goals and the ambitious commitments to limit global warming enshrined in the Paris Agreement.[4] "Transformation to healthy diets by 2050 will require substantial dietary shifts," says Professor Walter Willett MD, of the Harvard TH Chan School of Public Health, and co-chair of the EAT-*Lancet* Commission. "Global consumption of fruits, vegetables, nuts and legumes will have to double, and consumption of foods such as red meat and sugar will have to be reduced by more than 50%. A diet rich in plant-based foods and with fewer animal-source foods confers both improved health and environmental benefits."

Put simply, if you imagine a plate half filled with fruits, vegetables and nuts, and the other half filled mostly with wholegrains, plant proteins (such as beans, lentils and pulses), unsaturated plant oils and, optionally, modest amounts of meat and dairy, with limited added sugars and starchy vegetables, this is what a "saving the planet" diet looks like – and it could prevent millions of premature deaths every year worldwide.

It's clear there are myriad reasons for eating more plant foods, but do we need to give up meat completely? Many of us have been brought up believing that meat makes us strong, but it's not essential for a healthy diet in the way that vegetables are, and protein-rich foods also include beans and pulses, tempeh, tofu, nuts, seeds and grains such as quinoa and buckwheat.

One of the problems with meat and dairy products is that many people simply eat far too much – and often the cheap, intensively produced, processed varieties – at the expense of more nutritious foods. In an increasingly toxic food environment, where many of the most fashionable, accessible and affordable foods are ultra-processed products, it's especially important to focus on the real food heroes.

There is a wealth of scientifically backed evidence that suggests that the more red and processed meat you eat, the more likely you are to experience poor health. Studies have shown that even moderate intake of red and processed meat increases your chances of developing bowel cancer.[5] The problem may not be confined to cancer, unfortunately. A recent study looking into the effects of eating red meat and poultry on 25 non-cancerous illnesses that most commonly lead to hospital treatment in the UK, including heart disease and diabetes, found that people eating meat regularly (three or more times a week) were more at risk than those who ate meat less regularly, even after taking into account lifestyle factors, such as exercise, alcohol consumption and body mass index.[6]

On the flip side, while the EAT-*Lancet* report recommends a substantial global decrease in meat intake, the focus has mostly been on quantity rather than quality. Simply replacing meats with the highest carbon footprint, such as beef and lamb, with cheaper white, lean meats, such as mass-produced, battery-farmed chicken, is not the answer – for the planet, for people or animal welfare. If you're keen to cut down on red and processed meats for health reasons, then you should choose more nutritious, more humanely produced and more sustainable alternatives, or you are simply swapping one problem for another.

While you are making the transition to a plant-centred diet, or if other family members are not joining you on this journey, try to keep in mind the mantra that "meat is a treat". Meat is not something any of us need to eat every day, but occasionally eating small amounts of high-quality unprocessed meat (and other animal products) – which means locally produced products from regeneratively or organically reared, grass-fed, free-range, high-welfare animals that haven't been raised on deforested land – has a lower environmental impact and does provide beneficial nutrients. Yes, it is going to be more expensive, and rightly so, but if you are eating it far less often, the benefits for your health and that of the planet are worth it.

I realize that recommending people eat even small amounts of meat is not what the vegan community wants to hear, especially from an animal welfare perspective. But I believe being realistic and encouraging people to take this journey at their own pace pays dividends in the end. In my experience those who start meat-reducing, gradually come to find it less and less appetizing and digestible and soon find they rarely, if ever, buy it anymore.

So, let's reframe meat and dairy reduction in a positive way – it's not a sacrifice but an opportunity to make more space on your plate for a greater diversity of delicious plant foods, which will promote a longer, healthier life, for us and the planet.

# GROWING THE FOOD OF THE FUTURE

Eating more plant foods on a community, national and global level is a tremendously positive way to make a substantial impact on climate change, but if we want to eat a more diverse range of plant foods, we need to grow them too. While some of us may like to forage for wild food and grow some of our own fruit and veg, most people in wealthier nations predominantly eat cultivated produce from intensive farming systems.

One of the reasons that growing in your own back garden – or allotment or community space – is so important for living plantfully is that when you start to nurture plants yourself, especially edible varieties, you gain a deeper appreciation and understanding of what goes into producing even one bunch of carrots or punnet of strawberries.

Most of us are completely disconnected from how our food is grown, and in many ways, agriculture is also strangely disconnected from our health needs. If we wanted every person in the UK to consume even the minimum of five portions of fruit and veg a day, for example, we don't grow enough in this country to provide that. It makes little sense that what we produce is so disassociated from the food that is best for us to eat.

From a health and planetary perspective, our aim should be to grow a wider range of plant foods. In the UK, meat and dairy make up only a third of the calories we eat, yet we use 85% of the available farmland for feeding and rearing livestock, including growing crops for animal feed (although a lot of feed is also imported). It's a similar picture globally, with around three-quarters of the world's farmland used for livestock, yet only generating 18% of the world's calories.[7] It's an incredibly inefficient use of land, because growing plants for human consumption generates around 12 times more calories per hectare than using the land for meat production.

The problem with modern farming is that, over time, the range of produce grown commercially on a global scale has become narrower, which has had a knock-on effect on the diversity of our diet and created a less resilient food system, leaving us increasingly dependent on a limited range of crops, many of which are not terribly nutritious. Despite the thousands of exciting recipes we can now access online, there's a surprising lack of diversity in the human diet across the globe, as the UN Environmental Programme estimates that more than three quarters of the world's food comes from only twelve plant and five animal species. Kew Gardens reports that there are over 7,000 edible plant species, of which just 417 are currently considered to be food crops.[8] More than four billion people around the world mostly rely on rice, maize and wheat as their main source of nutrition. The irony is that many of these crops may not be resilient to climate change in some regions in the future, forcing farmers to embrace diversification eventually.

There's so much potential to grow many more delicious, nutritious, resilient crops, including plants such as fonio (a West African ancient grain), akkoub (a wild vegetable from the sunflower family) and chaya (a Mexican tree spinach), which some experts predict we could be using in our kitchens in the future. But it doesn't just have to be obscure new varieties, we could simply expand production of traditional crops we already know are good for us and beneficial for the soil, such as beans, pulses, seeds and ancient grains. The UK, for example, provides good growing conditions for highly nutritious plants including quinoa, barley, oats, broad (fava) beans, hemp seed, lupin, emmer, einkorn and chia, to name just a few, and every country on this planet has so much scope to diversify the plant foods they grow, which would have incredible benefits for biodiversity, soil quality and public health. But as consumers, we must do our bit by being more adventurous eaters, and show a willingness to embrace new foods to create enough demand and show producers that they can make a living from growing these alternative crops.

Although going plant-based for the planet is a positive choice, like all things to do with sustainability, making ethical choices can be a tricky balancing act, even with plant foods. Avocados are a good example of the murkier side of our global food system. I've seen so many vegan cookbooks full of recipes that use vast quantities of ethically troublesome ingredients, such as avocado, coconut oil and cashew nuts, in volumes that are eye-wateringly expensive too. It's important to face up to some of the ethical challenges these ingredients present. Is it right to show compassion for animals by rejecting animal products, and then consume foods that show no compassion for humans who are being exploited to produce them, or which are irreparably damaging the environment where they are grown? If we are going to eat more plants, then it's important that on a global level we are growing the right crops, in the right place, in the right way.

Clearing land to create vast avocado plantations leads to deforestation, which results in biodiversity loss, as food sources and habitats for local wildlife are destroyed. This type of highly intensive monoculture involves massive levels of chemical use, which pollutes and degrades soil quality and contaminates local water supplies. Then, there's the issue of water-guzzling. Global Food Security calculated that 25 million cubic metres of water (enough to fill 10,000 Olympic-size swimming pools) is needed to grow enough avocados for the UK market alone in just one year.[9] The prospect of drought and failed harvests when huge areas are so dependent on the success of one crop puts many people at risk of both water and food insecurity.

Sadly, the story of avocados is very similar to those of so many fashionable food crops, from soya to açaí berries. In some ways, it's hard to understand why monocultures have become so entrenched, when it makes so much more sense on every level to grow a greater diversity of crops, but larger farms focusing on one variety have proved to be more efficient, more productive and more profitable, as long as the quality of the food produced isn't a top priority – or taking care of the environment and the soil.

I know soil doesn't seem like the most exciting of subjects, but bear with me, because it's incredibly important to all of us. The microbiome of soil, which also contains trillions of bacteria, along with other types of microorganisms, helps to keep soil healthy. This goodness in turn supercharges the crops grown in the soil, providing them with nutrients that not only help them to grow, but also provide us with essential nutrients when we eat them. Just as our gut microbiome needs to be fed the right foods to ensure the good bacteria thrive, soil needs to be enriched with manure and organic plant matter to replenish the goodness and fuel the microbes. It's a beautifully balanced symbiotic relationship between microbes, plants and people, when allowed to flourish naturally.

Modern farming, however, appears to have been set up to do everything possible to destroy the soil, from ploughing and tilling it, which decimates the natural structure, to pumping it full of chemical fertilizers, while continuing to grow the same nutrient-draining crops year after year until every bit of goodness has been leached from the soil, and the only way to grow anything is to plough in even more chemical fertilizer. Tilling and chemical fertilizers are a significant source of the greenhouse gas emissions associated with agriculture, not just carbon but also methane and nitrous oxide, which are even more potent contributors to global warming.

John Cherry, a passionate advocate for regenerative farming on his farm in Hertfordshire, UK, and founder of Groundswell, an annual event to promote regenerative agriculture, says: "The soil is absolutely the most important thing for me as a farmer, and for everyone on the planet who needs to eat. We've abused our soil terribly and an awful lot of the excess carbon dioxide in the atmosphere has come from the soil and needs to be put back in there, which would make it much more fertile and help it retain more water and do all the things that good soil should do."

Using regenerative techniques, such as planting nitrogen-fixing herbal lays in the crop rotation, agroforestry and allowing livestock to graze the land to improve fertility with manure are natural ways to improve soil health, reduce dependence on chemical fertilizers and pesticides, and increase local biodiversity.

"We've all been conned by big pharma that we can buy soil fertility in a bag or a bottle, and farms have been ladling on fertilizers and growing amazingly high-yield crops since the end of World War II – but in the end it's ruined our soil," says John. "Now yields are decreasing and we have to spend even more on chemicals and put more on to get less back. We are making our soil worse and we can't afford to continue this way."

If the idealistic model of farming in the future is entirely organic, then perhaps the more realistic model to help us get there is regenerative farming, a looser philosophy with no strict rules, which can be introduced to farms in a more gradual, moderate way, ideally with going fully organic as the ultimate goal.

"Everything is interrelated – we can't just continue to grow food in this exploitative and damaging way led by chemicals and high-tech methods," says John. "Regenerative farming is a state of mind, a direction of travel rather than a destination, you could say. Nature does everything so well, we have to watch what nature does and try to follow in her footsteps."

# SIGNPOSTS

For more on:

- 🌱 Easy ways to eat more plants, *see* chapter 7
- 🌱 The benefits of growing your own, *see* chapter 3
- 🌱 Choosing ethical plant foods, *see* chapters 10 and 11
- 🌱 The impact of gut health, *see* chapter 7

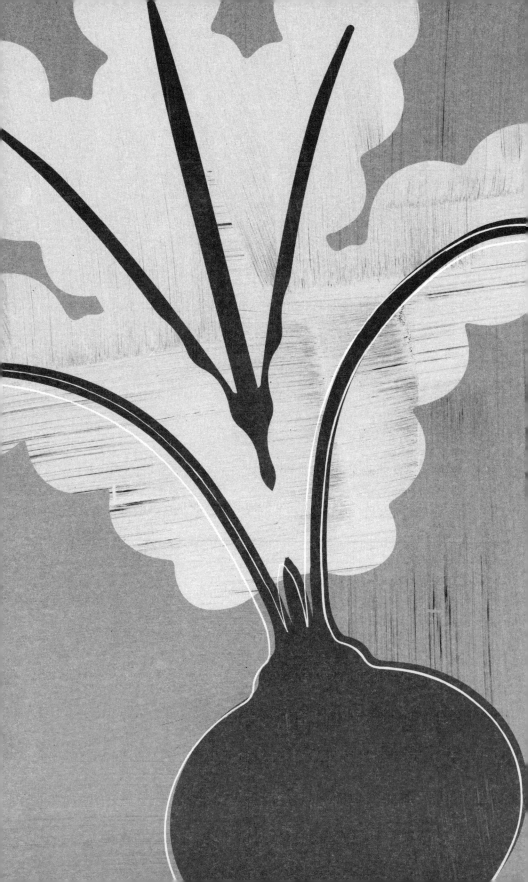

# GROW

Sow the seeds of a healthier, happier life by finding your green fingers and living more plantfully. Creating a closer connection with nature and the cycle of the seasons, growing is fun, inclusive and enhances your mental and physical wellbeing in myriad ways. Whether you want to nurture a veg patch to save on food bills, cultivate windowsill herbs to enhance your cooking or sprout microgreens to supercharge your nutrition, there are so many possibilities for enjoying growing on a scale that works for you.

Where flowers bloom, so do pollinators. Gardening enables biodiversity to flourish, bringing colour and vitality to our neighbourhoods, while trees bring their lush magnificence and almost mystical protective powers to our communities, purifying the air we breathe, supporting wildlife and making our world more beautiful.

# 3

# GROW YOUR OWN GREENS

"To forget how to dig the earth and to tend the soil is to forget ourselves."

Mahatma Gandhi

**THE GOAL:**
**TO CREATE A HOMEGROWN SALAD BAR**

**G**ETTING YOUR HANDS DIRTY IS GOOD FOR YOU. YOU KNOW HOW most children are magnets for mud? It turns out that their natural instinct to play in the dirt is a healthy one, as studies show that regular contact with soil is one of the best ways to develop a strong immune system and a flourishing gut microbiome into adulthood.

Lately, we've been hearing a lot about how the microbes in our gut keep us healthy, and thanks to some aspects of modern life, including spending too much time in sealed office spaces, over-prescribing of antibiotics, antibacterial cleaning products, pasteurized foods, children spending less time playing outside and the fact that most of us are completely disconnected from any kind of hands-on food production, we are not being exposed to the wide range and quality of microbes that our ancestors were.[1] Humans have enjoyed a symbiotic relationship with beneficial bacteria for many generations, but these protective microbes are increasingly being eradicated from our environment and our bodies, leaving our immunity compromised.

So how can gardening help redress the balance? We're getting used to the idea that "bacteria" is not such a dirty word, and now we know that gut microbes influence our immune system, it's not such a leap to believe that the trillions of microbes in the soil – where our food comes from – may also have a role to play. Heading out to the garden and getting your hands dirty on a regular basis can increase exposure to beneficial microbes and increase the diversity of your gut microbiome, boosting your immunity as a result.

Many people find that gardening boosts their mood, and there's plenty of scientific evidence to support this belief. My friend has an allotment that she calls her "happy place" – and it's not just because she keeps her secret stash of biscuits in the shed there. Keen gardeners, especially those new to growing, often talk about the transformative effect on their outlook on life, and this is partly due to simply being around nature and green spaces, which we know enhances wellbeing and is especially beneficial for people living in built-up urban areas. The impact on people can be so powerful that some doctors are now "prescribing" gardening for patients with conditions such as mild depression, anxiety or even loneliness. Often known as social and therapeutic horticulture, research suggests that patients prescribed "lifestyle" solutions often require less medication and need to access fewer medical services to manage their conditions. However, we also need to be careful not to medicalize nature – a recent study suggested that for people with mental health issues, feeling pressure to spend time outdoors can undermine the potential emotional and wellbeing benefits.[2]

But if you can find something that sparks joy, this provides all the motivation you need to keep doing it. A side benefit of spending time working on a community garden or allotment is making friends with like-minded growers over a cuppa and a chat by the shed. A flourishing new social network plays a huge part in helping people get outdoors for some fresh air and exercise, and the social side is just as important for wellbeing as a flourishing veg plot.

You may think you don't have time for gardening, but growing veg is good for busy people, as it is both mindful and practical. It helps to manage stress levels, enabling you to focus on the tasks at hand, while pushing any worries to the back of your mind for a while – or providing space and time to reflect on them in a peaceful, neutral environment – and you get a tangible outcome, such as bulbs blooming in spring or a basket of veg to take home for dinner.

On the subject of veg, one of the most significant health benefits for those who grow their own is that they tend to eat a wider variety of produce, boosting their wellbeing with a diversity of nutrients and antioxidants, along with extra fibre to help their good gut microbes flourish too.

As if all that wasn't enough, it turns out that gardeners are quite literally planting and weeding themselves happy, as scientists now believe that friendly bacteria in the soil may lift our mood on a chemical level, by helping to stimulate "happy hormones". Numerous scientific experiments with a common soil bacterium – *Mycobacterium vaccae* – have revealed it has a mood-boosting effect, stimulating the release of the neurotransmitter serotonin into the brain. Impaired serotonin production can cause depression, so triggering the release of serotonin has a naturally anti-depressant effect.[3] Even without the beneficial microbes, when you have seedlings ready to be planted out, produce that needs harvesting or weeds that need digging up, you'll find you have a good reason to step outside every day, even if it's just for ten minutes, and it's such a great way to clear your head. There's always another email to answer or a boxset to binge watch, but if you get hooked on gardening, you'll make time for your patch because your plants depend on you, and it's always nice to be needed.

It's pretty exciting to think that simple, low-cost solutions such as digging your garden and eating more fruit and vegetables can have such profound benefits for health and wellbeing.

# AN ANTi-AGEiNG REMEDY

Even if you don't do any digging, working in the garden has a range of physical benefits, from increasing muscle strength and bone density to lowering cholesterol and blood pressure, and ultimately slowing the effects of ageing. It's even better for you than hitting the gym, as research shows that exercising in nature outdoors reduces stress and allows the brain to go into a more restorative mode, which is thought to increase levels of an enzyme called telomerase. This enzyme is believed to help regenerate DNA in our chromosomes, through a process of "telomere lengthening", which allows cells to divide without damaging their DNA and remain healthy for longer, reducing the risk of diseases such as cancer and dementia, and potentially extending life expectancy.[4]

## GOOD FOR YOU, GOOD FOR THE PLANET

You might be thinking that it's a little unappetizing to open a chapter on growing your own veg by talking about bacteria rather than all the delicious produce you can nurture and eat. But this invisible "army" is so essential, not just for living – but thriving. It's well worth understanding how gardening can be so good for you and why it's such an essential part of living plantfully, before you even sow a single seed.

Regardless of your motivation for doing it, to plant, nurture and harvest your own fresh vegetables and fruit, and eat them straight from the vine or earth, is one of the most rewarding things you can do. It's amazing to think that an unassuming little seed can turn into a lush plant laden with courgettes or a huge rotund pumpkin, and the more you experience the incredible alchemy of growing for yourself, the more addictive it becomes. Each season you want to grow more and better.

You'll also find that growing something yourself – and I think this is especially true of growing edibles – is the best way to reconnect with seasonality and the natural life cycles of plants. In a world where we can buy raspberries or asparagus at almost any time of the year at the supermarket, eating seasonally is fundamental to living more sustainably. Your tastebuds will also enjoy a great awakening, as a freshly plucked peapod or strawberry tastes miles better than anything that's been transported in a refrigerated truck, and took a week to get from farm to fork. Amazing flavour, above all else, is a brilliant reason to grow your own.

It's not just flavour that's at its peak in freshly harvested homegrown veg – the vitamin, mineral and antioxidant content of fruit and vegetables also starts to tail off surprisingly sharply from the moment of harvest. There's a relatively long lead time between crops being picked to when they reach the supermarket shelf, and then they may be stored in your fridge for a few more days. The nutritional content is depleting all this time, so picking something fresh from the allotment or garden and eating or cooking it immediately is going to be tangibly better for you than anything you can buy in stores.

Studies have shown that vegetables can lose 15–55% of their vitamin C within a week of being harvested, while spinach can lose 90% in the first 24 hours. Perhaps more worrying than what is lost from our store-bought produce, are the unwanted extras added to it. A huge bonus of GYO is that your fruit and veg won't be tainted by the huge arsenal of chemicals typically used to grow veg commercially, something that Lucy Hutchings, gardener, author and founder of @shegrowsveg, says only really hit home for her when she started growing her own veg.

"There are so many benefits directly related to growing your own vegetables, beyond the benefits of a life filled with plants," she says. "For example, when I try to grow cabbages in my garden, they practically get devoured to a stump by the myriad creatures that want to eat them. I have to nurture them like precious commodities for them to have any chance of reaching the plate. So, when I drive past a vast field of enormous, pristine cabbages, I know there is no way that can happen without a huge amount of chemicals. The sheer volume of chemicals used to mass produce vegetables is terrifying. Growing your own means you can have complete confidence in the provenance of your food, which is really rare these days because most of the time we just don't know where our food has come from or what's in it."

The fact is that while the chemical pesticides used by farmers have been deemed safe for use on food crops individually, there is growing evidence that the cocktail effect of using dozens of different types together could make them more harmful, and not just for bees and biodiversity. Some foods have been found to contain up to 25 different pesticides in a single item[5] and many have links with diseases such as cancer, while others are endocrine-disrupting chemicals, which means they affect hormones and fertility. We don't yet fully understand the long-term health implications from this toxic accumulation, so the more you can do to reduce your intake of intensively produced food, the more you reduce any potential risks.

As an added bonus from a sustainability angle, homegrown organic produce also has no food miles and no single-use packaging, and while global food production produces 30% of the total greenhouse gas emissions,[6] the carbon impact of homegrown veg is negligible. It might feel like a small thing growing a few tomato plants, but if everyone grew just one thing to eat, that would soon become a lot of things *not* intensively farmed, sprayed with chemicals, transported or wrapped in plastic, which adds up to a very positive change on a national level.

Looking at the bigger environmental picture, the more people start growing their own produce, the more it helps to reduce our collective exposure to chemicals, builds a more resilient food system, improves soil quality and boosts biodiversity. Replacing just a fifth of store-bought food with homegrown could save around 30kg (66lbs) of carbon emissions a year per person on average.[7]

Plus, when your plot starts to get productive, you also save a lot of money.

## IS GROWING YOUR OWN EASY TO DO?

I've read many, many articles and books about growing your own and the one promise they all seem to make is that growing food is "easy" to do. But I'm going to present a balanced perspective here, from the point of view of someone who has made a lot of mistakes growing veg.

Yes, it is easy in some respects. If you plant a seed in soil, it will almost certainly grow – nature is pretty amazing that way. But the quality and quantity of what you produce can be hugely variable. I know this from experience, having harvested some disappointingly tasteless tomatoes and doll-sized new potatoes in the past. Even experienced gardeners get it wrong sometimes, but the beauty of gardening is that you can dig it all up, learn from your mistakes and start with a clean bed of soil to try something else the next season.

If you want to start with something simple – such as a few pots of herbs or salad veg – that's very achievable, even without much garden space, and you still get all the health and sustainability benefits. However, if your intention is to have a consistent supply of food and eventually become almost self-sufficient, it does take more space, some knowledge and plenty of trial-and-error. If you start to follow experienced amateur and professional gardeners on social media for inspiration, you'll see they often talk about experiments with varieties that didn't work or crops that were devoured by pests as much as their triumphs – at least the honest ones will.

Gardening is one of those "one size *doesn't* fit all" activities, because no two plots are identical, every gardener is working with their own unique mix of soil type and quality, climate and microclimate, space, aspect (for example being exposed to wind or sheltered by walls or fences), sun exposure, and the varieties they've chosen to grow, as well as the amount of time they have available to put into gardening. All of which means you just have to give things a try to see what works for you.

If you're worried that growing your own means your back garden will look more like an allotment than a place where you want to host a barbecue, there's no reason that a garden that grows fruit and veg has to look utilitarian. "I've always been an advocate for approaching growing edibles in the same way as flowering plants," agrees Lucy. "People often think they have to take a rather municipal approach with everything planted in neat rows in square beds. But a lot of veg plants are very beautiful and if you approach them in the same way you would ornamental plants, considering height, texture and colour, you can create a polyculture garden with everything mixed together in a border, especially if you experiment with space-saving techniques such as arches and vertical growing for crops like squashes and beans. It looks really pretty and is just as productive."

In many ways, this kind of polyculture is a more natural style of gardening, as plants in nature don't grow segregated in rows of their own kind but all mixed up together in the conditions that suit them best. It's better for pollinators and a much healthier approach to avoid concentrations of problems such as pests and diseases. It's taking the idea of companion planting to the next natural step, and means you'll rarely have bare patches in your border to attract weeds, as your perennials will be there to take up the slack after you've harvested your annual edibles.

"There is a very blurred boundary between the two types of plant anyway, as many edible varieties were originally imported to be ornamentals, while many plants we grow as ornamental flowers are edible too," says Lucy. "It presents an exciting opportunity for people with less space, as you don't have to make the choice between a beautiful garden and a productive one."

# HOW TO GET STARTED

If those verdant allotments bursting with vibrant veggies you've admired on social media seem a little intimidating, I suggest starting with a very small and specific project. There are loads of lists of suggested veg to grow for beginners, including varieties that are less fussy and generally provide a good outcome. What you really need to grow is the food you eat most. Open your fridge, think about what you and your family cook with regularly, and have a go at growing it.

Having said that, one advantage of growing your own is that you can be more adventurous both on your plot and on your plate by trying out varieties that are either expensive or harder to buy because they're not widely grown commercially, such as yellow courgettes or purple tomatoes. Growing some interesting or rare veg varieties will not only add exciting flavours to your plate, but it will also boost the diversity of your diet, because every fruit and vegetable has its own unique mix of nutrients and phytonutrients.

If you're a beginner, setting an intention to grow specific ingredients for something that you enjoy making regularly – which could be creating your own "salad bar" (see below), ingredients for your daily smoothie, herbal teas or even homemade pesto – helps prevent the sense of overwhelm when you get started. Each year you can add something new to your pots or beds as your confidence grows – along with your crops.

## SALAD BAR PROJECT

Growing your own salad bar is a great starter project. Most salad veg is quick to grow, so you'll reap the rewards within weeks.

If you're trying to live more plantfully, then you'll undoubtedly start eating a lot more leafy greens, but salad is also a fantastic place to start from an eco perspective. Figures from WRAP, the UK's leading sustainability and food waste charity, suggest the UK alone throws away around 80,000 tonnes of lettuce and leafy salads every year. It's a crazy waste of the nutritional benefits this food could provide us with and the resources used to transport and grow it. Lettuce, along with other salad vegetables intensively grown for year-round supply, has significantly higher carbon emissions compared to field-grown vegetables – and all those single-use plastic bags end up in landfill too.

You could just grow leaves initially, or combine a few veg, herb and flower varieties in containers, perhaps starting with the following suggestions.

- **Cut-and-come-again salad leaves** – these are preferable to round lettuces as they can be continually harvested throughout the growing season.

- **Tumbling cherry tomatoes** – very easy to grow and useful for many dishes beyond salad. You can also freeze them whole to use in sauces through the winter.

- **Radishes** – these add a lovely peppery bite to salads and are delicious roasted too.

- **Nasturtiums** – these look pretty and the flowers, leaves and seeds are all edible. The leaves taste a little like rocket (and make a great pesto), but are so much easier to grow.

- **Bunching onions** (also sometimes called Welsh or Japanese onions) – like a perennial spring onion (scallion) these grow in a clump, so you can harvest some and they will keep going. They return again each year. Great for keeping in a pot and if they get very large you can divide the clump into two pots.

- **Garlic chives** – a very easy herb to grow. All chives can be snipped as needed and their pretty flowers are edible too.

# WATERiNG

Don't use mains water in your watering can or – worse still – a hose pipe. Install lidded water butts to capture rainwater, which saves you money on your water bills too. Techniques such as applying mulch, watering at dawn or dusk on hot days, and using drip trays under your pots (remove in winter/cold weather to avoid waterlogging) all help soil retain water.

# CONTAINER VEG FOR BEGINNERS

Fruit and veg can be grown in pretty much any container, such as a pot, bucket, growing sack or even an old baby's bath, providing there are holes in the bottom, plus some gravel or small stones to enable water to drain away. Fill up with peat-free compost and start planting.

- **Strawberries** – these sweet fruits do very well in containers, including window boxes and hanging baskets, with the added benefit that keeping the strawberries off the soil helps prevent them from rotting or being eaten by slugs. They need plenty of water and a weekly feed throughout the growing season and they love sun. If you can, move your container around the garden to help them catch the best rays all day.

- **Peas and beans** – these do brilliantly in larger containers. Try peas, runner beans, French climbing beans, or pretty borlotti (cranberry) beans (which are great for drying). Grow them up an arch or make a "teepee" with four garden canes tied at the top for them to climb up; plant two or three beans at the bottom of each stick.

- **New potatoes** – These are fun to grow in a purpose-made potato growing bag. Start by "chitting" your seed potatoes – just pop them in an open egg box in a cool, light place, until the shoots are about 2cm (¾in) long – then sit them at the bottom of the growing bag, on 15cm (6in) of compost, and add just enough compost to cover them. Every time you see shoots poking through, add another layer of compost, until you reach the top of the bag. Let the foliage keep growing (they get quite big!) and dig up your spuds once the bushy leaves die down a bit.

- **Squashes** – all kinds of squash, pumpkins, marrows and bush courgettes (zucchini) can also be grown in pots or a planter if you choose the right varieties. Start a few off from seed and plant out the strongest-looking seedlings of each type. They will also happily crawl along the ground or grow up an arch or trellis if you buy a trailing variety – they'll need support as they get bigger. Unusual varieties, such as acorn or patty pan squash or yellow courgette, are really fun to try.

- **Chillies** – fresh chillies will spice up your cooking. They can be grown from seed indoors from early spring and then planted into pots outside after the risk of frosts has passed, in a warm but sheltered position. They don't need a lot of attention, other than watering little and often, and a weekly feed from when they flower. Pinch out the growing tips when around 20cm (8in) tall to encourage bushier growth. Choose your chilli variety carefully – there are many types from mild to super hot, depending on your taste.

# NO-DiG GARDENiNG

Soil has a whole ecosystem of organisms and microorganisms (which include microbes, protozoa, algae, mites, earthworms and larger earth-dwelling insects) that are already doing everything necessary to make it fertile, and it works perfectly without any intervention from you. Mycorrhizas are beneficial fungi, which thrive by taking sugars from plants. In return, they provide moisture and nutrients gathered from the soil to the plants. Turning soil over and slicing through it destroys this supportive network of beneficial fungi. As a result, gardeners are increasingly retiring their spades and adopting a no-dig approach.

Digging damages the structure of your soil, so weeding should be done by hand or using a hoe on the surface. Spread a mulch onto the surface of your garden once or twice a year and let the microorganisms create beautifully healthy soil for you. It's one of those rare situations in life where doing less work reaps more rewards.

# GARDENING TERMS DEMYSTIFIED

You've probably heard a few terms being used to describe different approaches to gardening or techniques, so to help you navigate what's what, here's a quick guide.

## PERMACULTURE

A sustainable, holistic approach to growing that aims to create gardens that have the diversity and resilience of a wild ecosystem. Permaculture is an overall philosophy not a single technique – it incorporates a variety of sustainable methods and ideals within it, such as no-dig gardening or growing organically.

## REGENERATIVE

An approach to growing that works with nature to enhance soil health, boosting biodiversity and minimizing waste of resources such as water. Regenerative can mean growing organically too (although not always) and includes techniques such as planting a mix of perennials and annuals to keep soil covered, planting trees, encouraging wildlife into the garden and introducing livestock such as chickens and ducks.

## ORGANIC

Organic growing is about nurturing plants and animals in the most natural way with minimal or no chemical inputs, using natural methods to feed the soils and livestock. It's a philosophy that embraces many sustainable growing techniques.

## BIODYNAMIC

Fans of biodynamic gardening say it's a natural extension of organic growing. It's an approach that champions chemical-free growing, biodiversity and soil health, but there's a spiritual angle to biodynamic growing, as it focuses on tuning into nature, connecting more deeply with the rhythms of your garden to identify the best times for planting and harvesting. It also calls for the addition of "biodynamic preparations" to the soil and compost.

## HEIRLOOM OR HERITAGE VARIETIES

These two terms are often used interchangeably and refer to plants that are in their original form, which have not been crossed with other varieties (known as hybrids) to achieve qualities such as higher yield or disease resistance. Grown for hundreds of years for their flavour, heirloom veg often come in many colours, shapes and textures. They are very rewarding to grow, although you may have to search them out from smaller independent suppliers.

## SEED SAVING

Seed saving has become increasingly important as a means of preserving heirloom varieties for future generations and fighting back against the domination of hybrids created by commercial growers. The seeds from hybrid varieties cannot be saved as they may revert to their original state and may have a poor flavour or not even produce fruit. If you grow heirlooms, you can enjoy the satisfying and thrifty practice of saving seeds and growing them year after year. You can find out more about why seed saving is so important at https://www.seedsovereignty.info

# HOW TO MAKE YOUR OWN COMPOST

One of the best ways to be an eco-friendly gardener is to establish your own compost heap to recycle garden and kitchen waste. Every 1kg (2lb 4oz) of homemade compost saves 0.1kg (¼lb) of carbon.[8] It also helps you to see exactly how much is being thrown away and makes you more conscious of food waste. Composting edible food still wastes the resources that went into producing it but doesn't increase greenhouse gas emissions, and it creates a product you can use to enrich your garden or veg plot. You can get really into the art and science of composting, but to get you started, here's how to do it.

- Buy a compost bin – there are some compact ones suitable for small gardens or, if you have a larger garden, you could build a structure from palettes or scrap wood.

- Place your compost bin on bare soil, on a level, well-drained spot.

- Worms should naturally take up residence to do the hard work of eating through the organic waste and turning it into liquid compost, but you can add extra worms if you like. You can buy worms for this purpose by mail order.

- Use the compost bin for veg and fruit peelings and waste, teabags, plant prunings, some grass cuttings (not too much as they can go slimy) – these are the "greens". The "browns" are scrunched up paper, cardboard and fallen leaves, which are slower to rot but add valuable fibre and carbon to the mix, and also create air pockets. Crushed eggshells add minerals. Don't include meat and dairy products (unless you have a digester type of composter), diseased plants, perennial weeds, dog or cat poo or nappies, which could lead to bad smells and unwanted visitors, such as rats.

- Keep a good balance between greens and browns so it doesn't get too wet or too dry and turn over the mixture regularly to keep it aerated.

- If you want a faster turnover of compost, try adding an enzyme-based compost activator, which should take just 10 weeks to produce useable compost.

In autumn (fall), don't overload the compost bin with too many fallen leaves. Instead, you can make leaf mould, another easy and sustainable way to enrich your soil. Simply gather the leaves and stuff them in a biodegradable bag, leave in a corner of your garden, and by spring you should have a moisture-rich soil improver that you can use as a mulch on your flower borders and veg beds.

# PEAT-FREE AND PLANT-BASED COMPOST

If you're buying compost, it's particularly important to always buy peat-free. Peat is the part-decomposed remains of mosses, mostly dug from lowland sphagnum peat bogs. When these bogs are drained, unique natural ecosystems are destroyed and the peat releases carbon dioxide. Left undisturbed, these peat bogs act as "carbon sinks" absorbing huge amounts. The planet has 10 billion acres of peat, holding more carbon than all the world's forests combined. You may not realize this but peat is a fossil fuel, and extracting it destroys one of the Earth's most important ways of storing carbon safely. Furthermore, we are using it faster than it can form – it takes 100 years to create just 10cm (4in) of peat.[9] Peat-free compost is now widely available – check labels carefully though, as terms such as "organic" and "eco-friendly" do not automatically mean the mix is peat-free.

Not all compost is vegan-friendly either. Many commercial compost mixes contain ingredients such as fish blood, bone meal, shell, chicken droppings, cow horn and manure. You may have to look beyond the standard garden centre bags to find brands that use only plant material such as coir, wood fibre and composted bark rather than animal products.

# HOW TO GROW WITHOUT "GARDENING"

If weeding and mulching really don't appeal or you don't have any outdoor space available, there are lots of other interesting ways to grow edibles at home. You may not get as many of the microbial or exercise benefits if you're not in contact with soil or being active outdoors, but you'll still enjoy the fun of growing food and the extra variety and nutrients in your diet.

Microgreens and sprouts are cheap and easy to grow indoors all year round in a small space, yet their nutritional impact is relatively substantial because they are so rich in antioxidants.

Both sprouts and microgreens are best eaten raw to preserve their goodness and flavour.

Sprouts are newly germinated seeds that are harvested before leaves start to grow. They can be grown hydroponically (without soil) and don't need light or air. You eat the whole thing and not just the shoots.

Microgreens are the adolescent shoots of almost any sprouting green vegetable or herb – from kale to rocket (arugula) and Swiss chard – that is harvested shortly after germinating, usually 2–4 weeks after sowing. They are usually best grown in compost (although can be grown hydroponically) and are tender and milder in flavour than the fully grown vegetable. You've probably grown microgreens at some point without even realizing it – garden cress, from the same family as mustard and watercress, with a similar peppery flavour, is a very common variety that almost every child has grown on kitchen paper at some point.

Here are some windowsill projects to try.

## 1 PEA SHOOTS

Great for growing in a small space indoors and throughout the year, pea shoots are one of the fastest-growing microgreens. Tasty and packed with nutrients such as vitamin C (ten times more than blueberries), they also provide plenty of plant protein. They will grow in just a couple of weeks, making them the perfect choice for those who like a quick result.

Buy a bag of dried peas (the ones sold for cooking) and soak a handful in cold water for 24 hours. Fill a container with peat-free compost (at least 5cm (2in) deep, with drainage holes in the bottom) and water it. Scatter the peas across the top. Cover with a thin layer of compost and water lightly again. Keep the soil moist (not soaking wet) on your brightest windowsill and in 2–3 weeks (depending on the temperature) you should have shoots about 6–10cm (2–4in) tall. Pinch off each shoot just above the bottom set of leaves and you may get a second flush of shoots. Add to salads, risotto or stir fries just before serving (to preserve nutrients and taste) for a burst of crisp, fresh flavour.

This same method also works with dried small broad (fava) beans, which produce a lovely beany-flavoured leafy shoot.

After harvest, put the roots and compost on the compost heap, or scatter onto the garden, and start afresh with your next batch.

## 2 GARLIC GREENS

There are lots of fun ways to grow something new from kitchen scraps, but this project is particularly appealing because it doubles up as a food waste solution too. We've all had a garlic bulb that's gone rogue – sprouting long green shoots because it's been hanging around for too long. Don't throw it away – use it to grow some tasty garlic greens.

Peel the outer skin off the individual cloves, and then place them in a small glass jar with the shoots pointing upward. You can use a couple of pebbles to stabilize them if necessary. Cover with around 1cm (½in) of fresh cold water (or enough to submerge the cloves but not the shoots) and keep on a sunny windowsill (changing the water every second day to prevent bacteria growing). Allow the shoots to reach at least 10cm (4in) in height for the best flavour, then snip off with a sharp knife. If you harvest just 5cm (2in) off the top, the shoots will keep growing, and you can continue harvesting indefinitely as long as you keep refreshing the water.

These garlic greens make a delicious garnish for salads, frittata, risotto, stir fries and pasta dishes.

## 3 BROCCOLI SEED SPROUTS

Most seeds can be sprouted – and they all pack a nutritional punch – but broccoli seeds are particularly nutritious because they contain the phytonutrient sulphoraphane, a powerful antioxidant that has been shown to have cancer-fighting properties.[10]

All you need is a bag of broccoli seeds sold for sprouting and a very clean glass jar, either a mason jar with a strainer lid or a specially designed sprouting jar. If you're going to do this regularly, I recommend you get a sprouting jar because they make it so much easier – they are fairly inexpensive and will last for years.

Soak your broccoli seeds in a bowl of cold, filtered water overnight in a cool, dark place. Rinse them off and transfer to the sprouting jar. If using a mason jar, you'll need to prop it at an angle on its side to allow the water to drain out onto a plate with some kitchen paper on top.

Keep the seeds in a cool, dark place for a further 3–4 days, rinsing them 3 times a day. Rinsing regularly is very important to prevent harmful bacteria from developing.

After about 24 hours you should see some little yellow shoots forming. When the sprouts reach about 1cm (½in) in length, move the jar out into indirect sunlight to allow the shoots to green up for another day or so.

Give them one final rinse and they are ready to eat after about 5 days. They can be kept in a sealed container in the fridge for up to 5 days. They have a mild, spicy-ish flavour and are best eaten raw to preserve their nutrients – pop them in wraps and sandwiches, mix into homemade hummus and scatter onto salads.

# SIGNPOSTS

For more on:

- Gut health, *see* chapter 7
- Inflammation, *see* chapter 2
- Health benefits of nature, *see* chapter 1
- Planting for pollinators, *see* chapter 4
- Soil health, *see* chapter 2
- Farming and sustainability, *see* chapter 2
- Growing herbs, *see* chapter 4

# 4

# MORE THAN JUST A GARNISH

"Throughout our history, herbs have been the foundation of our medicine, a major component in the kitchen, and essential in the home. Quite simply, herbs are an indispensable part of our lives."

Jekka McVicar, *A Pocketful of Herbs*

**THE GOAL:**
**TO PLANT THREE HERBS AND FIND NEW WAYS TO USE THEM**

**T**HERE'S SOMETHING MAGICAL ABOUT HERBS.
Used for flavour, fragrance, nourishment and medicine, these aromatic plants have enhanced our wellbeing for centuries. The more you learn about herbs, the more you appreciate the ingenuity of nature in giving potent properties to such unassuming plants. You can't help but admire human ingenuity too, for finding so many ways to harness their powers.

We know from ancient Egyptian, Greek, Indian and Chinese writings that herbs have been used by many cultures over the centuries, for culinary, household and medicinal purposes. Previous generations fully understood the value of "living plantfully", and in the Middle Ages, most monasteries cultivated *physick* gardens as herbs were so important for making tonics and medicines in a pre-pharmaceutical age. In 1653, botanist and physician Nicholas Culpeper published his famous *Complete Herbal,* providing an illustrated "key to physic" of over 400 herbs, from adder's tongue to yarrow. While I'm not suggesting you start growing blessed thistle (for treating jaundice and bites from mad dogs) and mandrake (for expelling demons from sick people) unless you really want to, once you start living more plantfully, you'll find it fascinating to explore the deeper potential of plants in your life and the myriad ways they can enhance your wellbeing. When it comes to herbs, it seems our elders and ancestors really did know a thing or two about how to exploit their powers, knowledge gained mainly from trial and error in using them for cures over the centuries. While many herbs have interesting traditional medicinal benefits – for example, people chewed parsley for fresh breath or drank lemongrass tea for headaches – scientists now know even more about their health-promoting potential, and their powers go far beyond easing niggling everyday conditions. Herbs such as parsley, oregano, chamomile and mint contain polyphenols known as flavonoids. Many of these are antioxidants and can suppress inflammation in the body that is believed to contribute to the development of conditions such as type-2 diabetes, heart disease and cancer. Flavonoids are also found in other plant foods, such as onions, kale and citrus fruits. For optimum health, it's a good idea to get your plant powers from a wide variety of sources, including herbs.

# AN EXPLOSION OF FLAVOUR

Antioxidants aside, we may not primarily enjoy herbs for their health benefits these days; instead, we are drawn to their potent flavours in the kitchen. Few of us would brew a cup of rosemary tea to combat a hangover, but we may still enjoy the flavour of rosemary-roasted parsnips. While it may never occur to us to make a love potion with coriander (cilantro), as they did in the Middle Ages, the stems and leaves of this ancient herb really bring out the flavour of curries, from Thai to Indian varieties. Herbs also work beautifully in desserts, tempering sweetness in recipes such as basil ice cream, mint chocolate cake or bay-infused panna cotta.

While many countries have herbs that have become a trademark addition to their cuisine – such as tarragon in France or the Scandinavians' use of dill – thanks to global trade, over the centuries herbs have crossed borders and found their way into all kinds of dishes around the world. The vibrancy and versatility of herbs is part of their charm and makes them cosmopolitan guests at any gathering of ingredients.

Most of us tend to use herbs like a garnish or seasoning, only adding a small scattering to food. But soft herbs can be treated more like a vegetable or salad leaves, added in abundant quantities to dishes to boost flavour and goodness. Many cuisines have some form of herb salad, from the Vietnamese combination of fresh mint, coriander (cilantro) leaves and crunchy stems, often served with red chillies and lime juice and served as a side dish, to an authentic Levantine *tabbouleh*, the star ingredient of which is flat-leaf parsley – even though it's more often made as a predominantly bulgur-wheat salad, with more grain than parsley.

Herbs are flavour bombs, and we should all be much more generous in our use of them, as they add such an explosion of flavour to dishes. It's especially important when you take ingredients with a strong and distinct flavour out of your cooking – such as meat or cheese – to find healthy ways to pack that flavour back in and make recipes taste just as satisfying without them. Many plant-based alternatives, such as beans or tofu, may be nutritious but they're best when infused with dynamic flavours, and herbs and spices are an easy way to add some extra oomph.

When you go to a really good restaurant, the flavours always seem heightened, and often so much more vibrant than the food you cook at home. Take your cooking cues from the best professional chefs, who use herbs and spices abundantly to enhance the natural flavours of their ingredients. But it's not just a cheffy thing to do – if you're moving toward a plant-centred diet, herbs are your secret weapon for adding extra flavour and nutrition to your food, and they are far better for you than using shop-bought sauces and dressings or adding lots of salt.

If you're not already using herbs liberally in your cooking, you really are missing a trick as they are such an easy way to make every dish next-level delicious.

# HERBS VS SPICES

Herbs and spices are both valued for their powerful flavours, nutritional benefits and medicinal properties, but herbs are derived from the leafy parts of plants, while spices are ground from seeds, roots or woody parts of plants. Although spices are also a wonderful way to bring incredible flavours, nutrients and antioxidants into your cooking and should be used liberally, this chapter focuses on herbs as they can be grown in our gardens, whereas most spices cannot be easily cultivated at home and are almost always imported from warmer climates.

# FROM TIRED TO THRIVING

If your only contact with herbs is with supermarket varieties, you could be forgiven for thinking that they're often a little disappointing. How often have you bought a bright leafy pot of basil with a heavenly aroma, placed it on the kitchen windowsill, but then had to throw away a shrivelled specimen with blackened foliage less than a week later? Yet it's not your fault it died. Supermarket herbs are simply not grown for longevity. They are grown to look good on the shelf for a short while to entice customers, and that's why it's best to use potted supermarket herbs as quickly as possible, ideally within a couple of days of buying them. Don't assume that because your potted herb is a living plant that it will survive much longer than a packet of cut herbs.

Supermarket herbs are one of the most thrown-away foods, along with bagged salad leaves, with some figures suggesting we throw away over half the fresh herbs and leaves we buy, yet they also have one of the highest carbon footprints as most are grown in greenhouses that use tremendous amounts of energy to heat them. To compound the issue, they often come in plastic pots with a plastic wrap to protect the delicate leaves. So, if you are buying supermarket herbs, firstly try to buy varieties in plastic-free packaging if possible – some retailers are switching to paper pouches for living herbs, which you can then place in your own pot at home – and secondly, use them quickly to prevent waste.

Usually grown from seed, the young plants produced for large retailers are often packed too tightly together in one pot, and overcrowding is the main reason they don't thrive. Dividing them into smaller clumps and potting them separately gives them space to grow (*see* box for tips). Keeping them outdoors from the spring to autumn (until the first frost) may also help them live longer. This technique doesn't always save them, but if it does work you will have more plants to grow on for yourself or to give as gifts. Not bad for a potted herb that probably didn't cost that much in the first place.

# DiViDE AND CONQUER

Try this simple technique for helping your store-bought potted herbs to survive and continue to produce fresh herbs for many months – or for evergreen varieties, years.

1. Water the plant well and then squeeze the pot to loosen the rootball, and gently ease it out of the pot.

2. Gently tease the rootball apart with your fingers to make two or three individual plants, each with a decent set of roots.

3. Replant each one into its own pot (with holes in the base and a saucer for drainage), fill with multipurpose peat-free compost and push down on the compost to bed the plant in firmly.

4. Cut back most of the herb foliage above lower buds and shoots (and use in your cooking). Place the pots in a sunny, warm spot (especially important for basil), such as a kitchen windowsill, and they should continue to produce new shoots all season. Evergreen shrubs such as rosemary, thyme and sage can be divided in spring and grown on in separate pots, then planted outside in your herb bed or larger containers.

5. A regular dose of organic plant feed during the growing season will help keep potted herbs in tip-top condition.

# GOOD FOR YOU, GOOD FOR THE PLANET

To enjoy herbs at their best and freshest, growing your own is the way to go. Herbs grown from seed and forced to grow quickly in a greenhouse to supply a supermarket just don't have the depth of flavour of garden herbs, while woody varieties like thyme and rosemary need to be grown from cuttings to achieve a peak of flavour.

Thankfully, many herbs are easy to grow, requiring very little effort, so they suit lazy gardeners and busy people alike. If you're not sure growing carrots and spuds is for you, focusing on herbs will make you feel like a gardener without all that plot preparation and mulching. Compact, pretty and aromatic, most herbs grow beautifully in containers or vertically on "living walls", making them perfect for beginner gardeners or anyone with limited growing space or even no garden soil at all.

From a sustainability perspective, growing your own is undoubtedly the best option, reducing the planetary resources invested to grow the plants, the food miles and packaging, and finally the potential for food waste. But most importantly, you can diversify the range of herbs you use, as wonderful varieties such as lovage, sorrel and chervil are simply not available to buy as they are currently not grown commercially. Interestingly, these are often the easiest to grow at home, while the most familiar herbs such as basil and coriander (cilantro) can sometimes be the most challenging to grow yourself.

If you really want to have a year-round supply of herbs, it's a good idea to get some plants established outdoors too, even if it's just a few pots outside your kitchen door. They may grow indoors, but they will thrive outdoors, and you can enjoy a greater variety of these gorgeous greens.

So, why not start by choosing three herbs and planting them in a windowsill box or patio pot, and see how they grow. I'm sure you've read many a newspaper or magazine article extolling the benefits of growing a herb garden and the beauty of this project is that you don't need to spend a lot to do it. Raid your recycling box for large yoghurt tubs or bean cans to use as planters. Wash them out, punch holes in the bottom for drainage and place them on old saucers. Small herb plants from a garden centre are usually far less expensive than showy blooms, depending on the size and rarity of the variety (and it's even cheaper if you use the technique suggested for nurturing supermarket potted herbs on page 66). When you see your little plants flourish and taste their fresh flavours in your cooking, I can say with confidence that you'll soon be hooked on growing more.

But which herbs to choose? If you don't currently use many herbs, versatile classics such as chives, flat-leaf parsley and thyme feature regularly in recipes and are good ones to start with. But really, the choice of herbs to grow should be guided by whether you love their flavours. Do you cook a lot of Italian classics such as pasta, pizza or pesto? Then basil and oregano should be on your list. If you love mixing up cocktails with all the trimmings in the summer or can't resist a zingy fresh salad, then mint is for you. Rosemary and thyme bring wonderfully strong, aromatic flavours to all kinds of dishes, while if you're a spice or chilli fan, coriander (cilantro) brings a sharp freshness to so many cuisines, from Asian to Indian and Mexican dishes.

With a little love, perennial herbs such as rosemary, oregano, sage and chives will make themselves at home in your garden, providing a bountiful source of flavour for your cooking for many years. For a windowsill indoors, you may find the following annuals are a better choice. With all these annual herbs, don't forget to save some leaves to freeze or dry for use in winter (see storage tips later in this chapter).

## WATERING

Don't over-water herbs and ensure they are planted in deep, well-drained pots. Many originate in hotter, dryer climates so they don't need too much water and thrive best when very slightly neglected. Basil, in particular, does not enjoy having wet feet at night.

## BASIL

To grow: This aromatic annual grows easily from seed but keep it indoors on your sunniest windowsill until the warmer months, as it really doesn't like the cold and won't survive a frost. In the summer, you can pop it outside in a container in a sunny spot and it should flourish. Water and feed regularly (but don't let the soil get soggy) and you'll find one packet of seeds sown at intervals will keep you in fresh basil for months.

To harvest: If you pinch off the top of the plants so they don't flower, they will continue to produce all season. Avoid picking individual leaves but snip off side branches where they join the stem, and this will encourage a bushier plant with larger leaves.

## CORIANDER (CILANTRO)

To grow: Coriander is divisive – people seem to either love it or hate it. If you aren't keen on it fresh, do give it a second chance in cooking, because coriander becomes something else entirely when added to curries, bringing a fresh, balancing note when paired with rich, smoky spices and the heat of chillies. Coriander is an annual like basil and is usually best grown from seed at regular intervals to ensure a steady supply. The growing seedlings like plenty of space and water.

To harvest: Coriander needs to be picked regularly by pinching out the tips of each upright stem when they reach about 15cm (6in), as it bolts to seed quickly in hot weather – although this means it may self-seed new plants if it's in your border, giving you a longer harvest. Like basil, it won't thrive in winter even indoors, so dry or freeze it while you can.

## MINT

To grow: A great one for anyone a little nervous of gardening, mint is virtually impossible to kill. It will be happy in a container both indoors and outdoors all year round, or in a hanging basket – and although it loves sunshine this perennial survives the winter by going underground. It can be grown from seed, from a cutting or by dividing a mature plant. It's invasive and can grow pretty large, so if it's going in a border, plant it inside a sunken container to tame the roots.

To harvest: Mint needs to be pruned regularly so trim with abandon and enjoy it in cocktails, teas, salads, with fruit such as melon and strawberries, and in smoothies.

## FLAT-LEAF PARSLEY

To grow: You can grow parsley from seed, but it takes a while to germinate, so you might prefer to buy a plant for immediate rewards. It's very low maintenance; just keep it watered and place in a sunny spot.

To harvest: Cut single leaves or branches lower down on the stem. With a fresh, almost grassy flavour, flat-leaf parsley can be chopped finely and added to almost any dish, from grain salads to new potatoes, soups, veggie burgers, salsa, roasted vegetables, risotto and pasta.

## PROPAGATE YOUR HERBS

Many soft-stemmed herbs can be grown in water, and this is another way to propagate more plants from your supermarket herbs.

Take a nice healthy cutting from the main plant, place it in a clear glass or jar of water on a sunny windowsill and watch as it grows roots. Change the water regularly until you see the roots appear, then leave it until they reach around 5cm (2in), when it can be carefully planted in soil in a pot.

Try this with herbs such as mint, basil, coriander (cilantro), oregano and lemon balm. This is a fun growing activity to try with children too.

# BEGINNER AND BEYOND

When you've got some classic kitchen windowsill herbs going, you might like to move on to growing more unusual varieties in your garden. Judith Hann, former presenter of the BBC's *Tomorrow's World* programme, the former President of the Herb Society and author of *Herbs*, a beautiful cookbook and guide to using these wonderful plants, has devoted the last 25 years to nurturing her herb garden in the Cotswolds. If you're looking for an easy and enjoyable project with instant rewards, Judith says planting an outdoor herb garden is so satisfying.

"Herbs are the easiest plants to grow. I'd recommend them to beginners or to people who don't have the time to water and tend their garden every day," she says. "They like Mediterranean conditions, poor soil, little water, they really need so little maintenance. The salad herbs like rocket (arugula) do need watering more often, but most herbs need much less work than flowering plants.

"I think the appeal of growing herbs for most people is that you get an instant reward. Unlike vegetables, you don't have to wait for them to mature. Herbs can be left to their own devices until you need them, which means they are very economical, there's no glut like you get with fruit and veg when everything is ready to harvest at once and then you struggle to use it all up. I may grow over 150 varieties of herbs now, but I always say that actually you don't need that many herbs to have a massive flavour impact on your cooking."

# JUDITH'S TOP 3 UNUSUAL HERBS TO GROW AT HOME

### Lovage
I always suggest people grow lovage. You can't buy it as a cut herb in stores in the UK, but you can buy it as a plant from a garden centre or a nursery. Once you've got one, you've got it forever; I've got a 2.5-m (8-ft) run of it growing on the south side of my greenhouse. It has a wonderful, spicy, celery taste.

*How to use it:* Lovage soup is just so simple – make it with lovage leaves, maincrop potatoes, onion and garlic, with maybe some plant-based yoghurt stirred through once it's blended. It has the most deliciously unusual, subtle flavour.

### Chervil
Another favourite is chervil, which has the aniseed taste of tarragon and looks beautiful on the plate. It's an annual, but I've only ever bought one packet of seeds. I let them flower and go to seed, and then sow the seeds and leave them to grow over winter. Even though the plant has feathery, delicate leaves, it will survive even under snow.

*How to use it:* Blend dairy or plant-based cream cheese with garlic and chervil leaves for a delicious topping for toast or jacket potatoes, or leave to chill then form into balls and roll in chopped chervil to serve on a cheeseboard. Chervil and cauliflower also work well together in soup.

### Sorrel
Sorrel is one of my most-used herbs, I couldn't live without it in the kitchen. Sorrel is a perennial and I've got a 5-m (16-ft) run edging my salad herb bed. Although the plants were put in over 20 years ago, they are still going strong, they are just fantastic. I grow some different varieties too, such as red-veined and buckler-leaf sorrels.

*How to use it:* I like to make salads with lettuce, sorrel and lots of herb flowers such as coriander and marjoram flowers, the petals of Japanese chrysanthemum and beautiful blue chicory flowers.

# HERBS FOR POLLINATORS

It's not just humans who love herbs – bees and other pollinating insects do too. If you'd like to enrich biodiversity in your garden, here are the top ten herbs for attracting pollinators.

1. wild marjoram
2. mint
3. fennel
4. borage
5. chives
6. rosemary
7. sage
8. hyssop
9. lemon balm
10. thyme

## PREPPING AND STORING

### PICK

For herbs in your garden or windowsill box – whether you are planning to cook with them or want to freeze or dry them – always try to pick them on a sunny morning when the plant's oils have the most vibrant flavour, ideally immediately before you plan to use them.

### WASH

Before using, wash your fresh herbs and leave them to air dry completely in a colander. Chopping wet herbs will result in a green mushy mess.

### CHOP

Ideally use a very sharp, large chef's knife or sharp mezzaluna. A blunt knife can crush rather than slice delicate herbs. Pile the herbs into the middle of the chopping board and, with one hand on top of the blade, chop backwards and forwards, with a gentle rocking motion.

## STORE

For cut herbs, the best way to store them is unchopped in a loose plastic bag in the salad drawer of the fridge. Some people recommend keeping the stalks in a jar of water as you do with flowers, but they will rot if left too long. These delicate plants are best used quickly while very fresh.

## FREEZE

Supermarket herbs wilt quickly, especially the cut varieties, so to preserve their freshness get into the habit of popping them in the freezer and using them straight from frozen, which preserves both flavour and nutrients. It won't preserve their attractive leafy look, so frozen herbs are not really suitable for your cocktail garnishes or salads.

To freeze, chop herbs and sprinkle on a baking sheet, then pop in the freezer. Once frozen, they can be bagged (this method prevents clumping). Alternatively, freeze in ice cube trays and top up with water. Once frozen, store in a bag. The cubes can be added to soups and stews, or other dishes where a little extra water won't affect the flavour.

To save them for dishes such as sauces and stir fries, chop finely or pulse in a food processor and freeze in ice cube trays with a little olive oil, which preserves their punchy flavours. Try freezing basil in extra virgin olive oil for adding to tomato-based pasta sauces, or rapeseed oil with rosemary for roast potatoes. You can also chop herbs into softened plant-based butter and freeze – chive butter is great for mashed potato or try minced garlic with parsley for garlic bread.

## PRESERVE

If you have large quantities of leftover herbs, making a quick pesto or salsa verde (see opposite) is a great way to preserve them for a few weeks in the fridge (drizzle a thin layer of oil on top and seal the jar) or pop them in the freezer. These can be used for pasta, for dressing salads or on pizza or flatbread.

Don't discard soft herb stalks, such as parsley or coriander (cilantro), as these can be chopped finely and added to dishes (they have tonnes of flavour) or frozen and added to homemade vegetable stock – simply strain out at the end with the other veg.

# HERBY DRESSINGS: TWO IDEAS

Herbs are the star ingredient in these two sauces, which are both so quick to make and can be used to add a flavour punch to so many dishes. They are a great way to save supermarket herbs at risk of going limp or shrivelling up, preserving their flavours to use with different dishes throughout the week, and can be adapted to whatever you have available.

## SALSA VERDE

*This classic herb dressing is traditionally made with basil, flat-leaf parsley and anchovies, but you can use any combination of herbs to make a vibrant green sauce. It can also be frozen to use later. It can be used to make a dip, or a salad dressing, or drizzled on soup, grains, new potatoes or roasted vegetables.*

**Serves 4 | Cooking time: 5 minutes**

### INGREDIENTS

**3 large handfuls of mixed soft herbs, such as coriander (cilantro), basil, mint, parsley, dill, chives, tarragon, sorrel or chervil** (leaves stripped from woodier stems for herbs such as oregano and marjoram)

**1 garlic clove**

**1 tablespoon chopped capers**

**2 tablespoons wine or sherry vinegar, or lemon juice**

**100ml (3½fl oz) extra virgin olive oil**

**salt to taste**

### METHOD

Either grind the herbs, garlic, capers and vinegar together in a pestle and mortar or whizz in a food processor. Then add the olive oil and season to taste.

## SAGE PESTO

*For a twist on a classic, switch basil and pine nuts for sage and walnuts. Sage pesto tastes wonderful drizzled on roasted butternut squash, stirred into spaghetti or even as a posh pizza sauce.*

**Serves 4 | Cooking time: 15 minutes**

### INGREDIENTS

**50g (2oz) walnuts**

**80g (3oz) fresh sage leaves** (or half sage and half flat-leaf parsley, for a milder flavour)

**1 garlic clove, crushed**

**100ml (3½fl oz) extra virgin olive oil**

**80g (3oz) Parmesan** (authentic Parmesan is always made with animal rennet, so you can opt for a vegetarian or vegan Parmesan-style hard cheese, or leave the cheese out)

**a generous squeeze of lemon juice**

**salt and freshly ground black pepper, to taste**

### METHOD

Lightly toast the walnuts in a dry pan, then remove from the heat and leave to cool.

Tip the cooled walnuts into a food processor with the herbs, garlic and extra virgin olive oil. Pulse until chunky, then add the cheese, if using, a generous squeeze of lemon juice and seasoning. Pulse again, adding a little more olive oil if too thick.

# DRYING HERBS

## WOODY HERBS

Woody herbs – such as thyme, rosemary, lavender and sage – are easy to dry by hanging in bunches. Tie the stems together and hang upside down outside to dry if it's warm (but not in direct sunlight), or indoors in a pantry or airing cupboard. When dried, store in airtight jars.

## SOFT HERBS

Soft herbs include basil, mint, lemon verbena, coriander (cilantro) and parsley. Pick the leaves and spread them over kitchen paper to draw out any moisture. Leave the tray near a sunny window (but not in direct sunlight) to dry for a few days, until they feel papery soft and look a little wrinkly. Store them in airtight containers separately or create your own herb mixes by combining different varieties, then simply sprinkle them into your cooking as needed. Keep dried herbs for a maximum of a year, as after this they start to lose their flavour.

**Quick Mix:** An Italian seasoning is great for pizzas or pasta sauces – mix equal quantities of dried basil, oregano, thyme, marjoram and rosemary, and add a little dried sage. Drying herbs concentrates their flavours so you won't need to add the same quantities as fresh herbs.

# PLASTiC-FREE TEA BREAK

With many tea brands still using plastic in their bags and packaging, you can brew a healthier, budget-friendly, eco-friendly cuppa with fresh homegrown herbs. Technically known as a tisane rather than tea, most herbs and spices can be used to make a soothing hot drink. Many of the best herbal tea brands have a premium price tag, so for the same cost of one fancy box of herbal tea that might last you a couple of weeks, you could buy a herb plant that will keep you supplied with fresh herbal tea for many months or even years, which is a pretty savvy investment.

## HOW TO MAKE A TISANE
### With fresh leaves
Simply pick a few fresh herb leaves (crush soft leaves gently in your hand first to release the oils), then pop into your teapot or infusing ball. Add just-off-the-boil water and infuse for a few minutes to your preferred strength, then strain and enjoy. Add honey or agave syrup for sweetness or a squeeze of lemon for freshness, if you wish.

### With dried herbs
As a guide use ½ teaspoon per ingredient for each cup of tea you are making and simply infuse them in a teapot (and use a strainer) or an infusing ball.

Some herbs are stronger in flavour than others, so it's best to play around with the balance of ingredients to find your perfect blend.

**Moroccan Mint:** One of the easiest and most prolific herbs to grow. You can grow standard garden mint or try varieties such as Moroccan (especially good for tea), peppermint or even pineapple mint. It also pairs beautifully with lemon thyme or rosemary and has long been used for its soothing effect on the digestive system. It also makes a great mojito.

**Lemon Balm:** Another very prolific herb that's probably best contained in a pot, unless you have a huge garden. Looks a little like mint but has a soft lemon flavour that tastes so refreshing as a tea. Believed to help mild depression and anxiety, lemon balm can be helpful for relaxation and to promote sleep.

**Rosemary:** This woody herb makes a delicious fresh tea and you can balance out the distinctive piney flavour with lemon or honey, or both if you prefer. Antibacterial and rich in antioxidants, rosemary has many beneficial properties, including enhancing mood and concentration.

**Note:** Remember to check the safety of any herbs you use for cooking or making teas or remedies, as they can be potent. This is especially important if you have any underlying health conditions, are taking medication or are pregnant or breastfeeding. For example, raspberry leaf tea, while harmless for most people, is not usually recommended during pregnancy as it softens the uterus.

## SIGNPOSTS

For more on:
- Inflammation, *see* chapter 2
- The benefits of growing your own, *see* chapter 3
- Foraging ideas, *see* chapter 12
- Planting for pollinators, *see* chapter 5
- Using herbs in natural cleaning products, *see* chapter 14

# 5

# LET'S TALK ABOUT THE BIRDS AND THE BEES

"After all, in truth, if all things are interdependently connected, as the wise ones throughout history proclaim, then we cannot consider ourselves as separate from the rest of creation. There is no separation between the garden and the gardener."

Ark Redwood, *The Art of Mindful Gardening*

**THE GOAL:
TO START WITH LAVENDER**

**A** **GARDEN THAT'S BRIMMING AND BUZZING WITH WILDLIFE** has more energy – it makes us feel more alive too. Maybe you don't think you're much of a gardener, but planting lavender in your garden – or on a balcony, in a courtyard or window box – can be the start of a journey to enriching biodiversity in your neighbourhood. Beautiful, fragrant and edible, lavender happens to be a favourite of pollinators, and that makes it a potential game-changer for nurturing a happier and healthier ecosystem. If you truly want to live more plantfully, you must start thinking about what you can do for nature and not just what nature can do for you. Of course, one of the richest rewards of getting into gardening is the colour and fragrance of beautiful blooms bringing joy to your space – and lifting your spirits – all year round. You'll soon be hooked, and will almost certainly find yourself planting more than lavender.

With culinary and aromatic qualities, lavender has a long history as a therapeutic herb. It was used by the ancient Egyptians as perfume and for mummification rituals, and the Romans for aromatic bathing. Lavender oil has long been treasured for its calming and soothing qualities, which is why it's often found in products such as pillow sprays, hand cream and bath soaks.

Lavender is loved by bees and butterflies, and you really don't have to be at all green-fingered to grow it; it can even be grown from cuttings taken from a friend's plant. There are many varieties to choose from, but in his wonderful book exploring biodiversity in our back yards, *The Garden Jungle*, Dave Goulson recommends *Lavandula x intermedia* as the most popular pollinator choice, based purely on observations in his own garden. However, based on observation in my own garden, most of my lavenders seem to be pretty popular with buzzing visitors in the summer, so don't worry too much about seeking out special varieties, as this can come with time and experience.

Growing your own vegetables is a wonderful thing to do, but if you're not much of a gardener (yet) or space is limited, it can be simpler to start with undemanding flowering plants. If you don't have a garden, lavender, along with many other kinds of flowering plants, will also thrive brilliantly in a pot or window box. Despite all the talk lately about wildflowers being best for pollinators, cultivated (organic) garden flowers are often just as attractive to insects.

A couple of plants in containers may not seem like much of a contribution, but as with all steps toward sustainability, a small change can make a big difference, especially if millions of people do it. As deforestation and development caused by agriculture, industry and population growth intrude into wild places across the globe, threatening wildlife habitats and biodiversity everywhere, even the tiniest green spaces we nurture at home become increasingly important. Gardens can represent up to a quarter of the area of a city, which means collectively they are hugely important for providing habitat, food and other resources for wildlife in built-up areas. Studies show that areas with lots of small gardens are just as good for wildlife as larger gardens.

# THREE LOVELY WAYS TO USE LAVENDER

Harvest when the lavender buds are beautifully purple, just before they open into flowers, as this is when they are at their peak fragrance. On a dry day, cut stems at the base above the leaves, and tie together in small bunches. Hang upside down to dry for 7–10 days in a cool, dry place, away from direct sunlight, over kitchen paper or a tray to catch any fallen buds. Once dried, arrange the stems in a vase for natural room fragrance or use to make wreaths.

### 1 Lavender Fragrance Sachets
Strip the lavender buds from the stems and sew them into little bags made from scraps of cotton or muslin fabric – these are a traditional way of fragrancing your linen cupboard and are a natural moth and insect repellent. Keep one under your pillow as lavender may promote better sleep.

**2 Lavender Tea**

Steep ½ teaspoon of dried lavender (*Lavandula augustifola* has a mild flavour suitable for tea) with ½ teaspoon of dried chamomile flowers or some fresh mint leaves in just-off-the-boil water for around 5 minutes, then strain and serve. Lavender tea reputedly eases tension headaches and calms anxiety.

**3 Lavender Sugar**

Dried lavender can be overpowering and "soapy" if used too liberally in recipes. Popping some dried lavender into a jar of caster (superfine) sugar (around 2 teaspoons per 1kg/2lb 4oz of sugar is a good ratio) infuses it with a subtle lavender flavour. You can use the sugar to make aromatic ice cream, lemonade, sugar syrup for cocktails, in baking, for making hot chocolate – or any dessert or cake that needs a scattering of sugar on top. The flavour tends to work particularly well with other herbs such as mint and thyme, and citrus like lemon and orange, especially in recipes such as shortbread, cakes and creamy desserts like ice cream or crème brûlée.

## SHOULD WE GO WILD?

By 2050, the UN predicts that 68% of the global population will live in urban areas,[1] so ensuring everyone has access to a green space of some kind, whether that's a private garden or a communal or community garden will become increasingly important. Partly inspired by spending more time at home during pandemic-related lockdowns, more people have been bitten by the gardening bug over the last few years, realizing that our outdoor spaces are not just somewhere to have the occasional barbecue and gardening is not just for the retired. The idea of gardening for wildlife – and consequently for the planet – has also sparked a plethora of ponds, bug hotels and bee-friendly planting, and this renewed passion for nature is really heartening to see.

There's also been a lot of talk about "rewilding" lately, which is a fascinating movement and something I certainly recommend you read more about, but true rewilding is not really something you can achieve in the average back garden. It's a progressive approach to conservation on a larger scale, which allows nature to take care of itself to repair damaged ecosystems and restore degraded landscapes. Sadly, most of us don't have space to introduce bison and beavers in our backyards or to plant a native oak forest, but we can certainly be inspired by the rewilding philosophy that we need to work with nature to restore broken ecosystems. In his book, *Back to Nature: How to Love Life – and Save It,* wildlife champion and TV presenter Chris Packham says, "While you and I can't reintroduce big birds and mammals, we can plant plants in our gardens and community spaces. We can introduce plants and trees locally and, if enough of us do so, we can start from the bottom up and install the fundamental building blocks of ecosystems ..."

Even on a small scale, the secret to creating a garden that is good for the planet and for wildlife is to plant something – anything – as even one plant is better than no plants at all.

Among all the talk of going wild in our backyards, the sustainable gardening trend seems to come with a whole set of new "rules". There are those who argue we should only plant native species, those who believe we should give up weeding and let things grow freely and, of course, there's the issue of "to mow or not to mow" (*see* page 85). But let's not suck the joy out of gardening with rules, putting more pressure on people to do the "right" thing for sustainability and biodiversity, when the main attraction of gardening is that it's enjoyable and reduces stress.

Helen Bostock, senior horticultural advisor at the Royal Horticultural Society (RHS), agrees. "There's a bit of a myth that your garden will only have value for biodiversity if you've specifically designed your garden to attract wildlife. There's a lot of evidence that just the practice of gardening, whether you know what you are doing or not, whether you deliberately garden with wildlife in mind or just want to make it look lovely for your own enjoyment, often quite by accident ends up being pretty good for wildlife anyway."

Many of our gardens do naturally mimic the natural landscape. For example, a typical garden may have a few shrubs, a few varieties of flowering plants and a tree or two, and all these elements provide resources that garden birds and insects love to find in their territory. "It's important to remember that we mustn't project how we see a green space onto how wildlife sees it, as they will have a different view entirely," says Helen.

The other reason not to get too hung up on rules is that our back gardens are so valuable for wildlife precisely because each space is managed in a different way. No two are alike, which makes them incredibly rich in resources such as food and habitats that help to promote biodiversity. We should also consider how our gardens are connected. People in the UK are particularly keen on fencing off their own little plots, whereas in North America back gardens are often much more open plots with just grass dividing the properties. But even if your neighbourhood is a patchwork of high fences, wildlife isn't necessarily inhibited by these barriers – with the exception of hedgehogs, perhaps – as birds, insects and small mammals don't care if it's your garden or your neighbour's; to them it's part of a larger territory. Although wildlife hasn't had a lot of time to adapt in evolutionary terms to an increasingly urbanized environment, it doesn't make as much difference to them as we might think.

This means there's no need to feel eco-guilt if you haven't got a pond or a bug hotel or a wildflower patch, or because you prefer a neat lawn to one that's left wild. The things you don't have in your garden, maybe the people at number 27 have. You don't need to tick every box to be a valid supporter of wildlife.

"If everyone had gardens that were a mirror image and we all followed the same garden blueprint that would actually reduce biodiversity," Helen says. "We need them all – the scrappier gardens, the ones with the neat lawns, the really overgrown ones covered in nettles and the ones with a vegetable patch."

So, if you don't like the idea of "rewilding", don't worry. Just do what you want to do and know that you're still making a valuable contribution.

The important thing is to get out there, live plantfully, do some gardening, and the more you do, the more you learn and engage with it, you'll naturally start doing things that encourage biodiversity.

# TO MOW OR NOT TO MOW?

It's easy to think of lawns as rather inert surfaces – somewhere to lay a picnic rug or play football. But research conducted by citizen scientists across the UK for the environmental charity Plantlife's "Every Flower Counts" survey revealed over 200 wildflower species thriving on British lawns. Together, all the flowers counted had the capacity to produce 23kg (50lb) of nectar sugar every day, with lawns able to support anything from 400 to 4,000 bees and other pollinators a day.

Based on the research, the charity now advises giving your lawn a "Mohican" cut – leaving some areas completely unmown to allow taller flowers to come into bloom, while cutting the rest of the lawn only once a month to a height of 2.5–5cm (1–2in). This allows the flowers that grow better in shorter grass to continue flowering throughout the season, putting out new blooms after each cut.[2] Find out more at www.plantlife.org.uk

## BEES ARE THE CHAMPIONS

Have you noticed that you can get everything from T-shirts to dish cloths with bee prints on lately? Bees have become something of a hero species for promoting biodiversity, and it's easy to understand why people connect with them. Every child learns that bees make honey and these charming creatures are often found buzzing across the pages of children's picture books. We connect with bees in a way we can't with creatures we see as creepy, slimy or pests, such as earwigs, slugs or wasps, and even as non-scientists we can understand the ways bees help us by pollinating crops

# DEFINING TERMS

The words "ecosystem" and "biodiversity" get used a lot lately, and while you probably have at least a vague idea of the definitions, it's worth clarifying exactly what they mean.

**Ecosystem:**

This is a geographic area where living elements such as plants, animals and other organisms, and non-living factors such as weather, rocks, humidity and temperature, work together to form a "bubble" of life.

Each element of an ecosystem depends on every other factor, either directly or indirectly, and even a tiny change in one element has an impact on others. For example, a change in temperature may change which plants can grow there, which then affects habitats and food sources for wildlife.

The Earth is covered in a series of connected ecosystems, which can vary in size and may be very small, such as a rock pool. Ecosystems covering a large section of land, sea or atmosphere with similar characteristics are known as a biome, and this could include a reef, a desert or a rainforest.

**Biodiversity:**

This encompasses all the species living in one area or ecosystem, which can be a small space such as a garden or the entire planet – including everything from the smallest bacteria to fungi, insects, birds, animals, trees, plants and humans.

The more trees and plants an ecosystem contains, the more species it can support by providing resources such as habitats and food.

we eat. So, when we read media reports that bees are endangered, it provokes an emotional response, even if much of our understanding about bees is pretty limited and often completely incorrect.

It's true that bees are the most important group of pollinators in the world – with around 20,000 species of bees worldwide – and they are at risk thanks to widespread use of pesticides, loss of habitat and diminishing availability of pollen- and nectar-rich flowers. Malnourished bees also have compromised immunity and are at greater risk of catching diseases. But interestingly, what most people think of as bees are honeybees, which are not endangered. The UN's Food and Agriculture Organization reports there are more than 90 million honeybee hives globally, and research from Kew Gardens in London reveals that the popularity of bees has fuelled a huge rise in the number of people keeping their own hives, which in combination with a reduction in pollinator-friendly habitat and a lack of understanding of how honeybees interact with other species, could be putting native bees at risk.[3]

In the UK alone, 270 native species of solitary bees and 25 of bumblebees are endangered, with some varieties near extinction living in isolated populations found only in one small geographical area. The best way to support pollinators is to take up gardening rather than beekeeping, which will support thousands of species including butterflies, moths, wasps, beetles and flies, not just bees.

The favouritism shown to bees is a brilliant illustration of how, with the best intentions but imperfect knowledge of how ecosystems work, we can cause more harm than good when we support one species over others. Champion species can be a useful entry point for understanding the importance of biodiversity, and while campaigns for activities such as feeding garden birds in winter and planting for pollinators are all very positive, we need to stop picking and choosing the wildlife that we support. It may sound a little hippyish, but we must rekindle a childlike sense of wonder of ALL the amazing flora and fauna in our world. Children have a pure love and appreciation for nature and wildlife; young people interested in conservation usually want to protect species simply for being an orca or a polar bear because they understand how marvellous it is to have these creatures in our world. But as adults, we often only relate to wildlife when we see it makes a contribution to our own lives; in effect we're applying a cost-benefit analysis to these creatures. Do we support protecting bees over less glamorous or useful creatures simply because they are a bee and we feel they belong here as much as we do, or are we more concerned with protecting our future food interests? I would argue both reasons are equally important.

We have such a superficial knowledge of how our ecosystems work and the role of the thousands of species within them, that it's a risky strategy to focus on the needs of a few. Even scientists still have much to learn about the complex interdependent relationships of everything from microscopic organisms up to apex predators within an ecosystem.

"It's quite naive of us as a species to think we can dispense with all these other species without consequences," says Helen. "However, maybe wonderful, relatable stories are the way to get the conversation started. Earwigs, for example, are not particularly well-loved, but they have tremendously good parenting skills. They really care for their young and protect them. People love to hear this fact about them and, for some people, human empathy is the best way to connect."

However we achieve it, we need to focus on the greater web of life and find ways to support the whole complex food chain, which may include species we think of as garden pests – because yes, we do need the slugs and wasps too – and we can't pick and choose what we want from nature because a healthy ecosystem needs everything working to be resilient. "If we only support species we see as attractive or useful then we risk losing this connectivity, the circle of life," says Helen. "The word 'ecosystem' can turn a lot of people off, but we must get across the idea that all living things are interdependent and even if we never see them, we still need them. Some things are too small for us to see the work they are doing - the microbes in the soil that keep it healthy, for example, or little springtails that eat algae from leaves - and by neglecting these we are doing ourselves an injustice and preserving only a tiny piece of the bigger picture."

# GOING NATIVE — OR NOT?

So, if we want to support a wide range of wildlife, what do we grow? And should we only plant native species? There are 80,000 plants listed in the RHS plant file alone, and we can't possibly know about every cultivated plant's individual contribution to our ecosystems and biodiversity. A quick scan online will reveal many "planting for pollinators" lists and they are all different, so it can be confusing. Not to mention that new discoveries are continually being made – nearly 4,000 species of plants and fungi were scientifically named for the first time in 2019 alone, according to Kew Gardens.[4]

As it turns out, plant variety is as important in our gardens as it is in our diet. Taking care of the very smallest inhabitants of your garden has the biggest impact for biodiversity, according to the results of a four-year research project at RHS Garden Wisley. The "Plants for Bugs" study discovered that a mixture of plants from different regions is best for pollinators, ideally with native plants combined with some exotic varieties to extend the flowering season and provide food for wildlife for longer.[5] The more flowers you can provide, the better. Although other insects such as ladybirds, caterpillars and woodlice tend to favour native and near-native species, the most important factor is to pack in as many plants as possible, including plenty of evergreens to provide winter habitats, as these bugs love densely planted coverage all year round. "Overall, what we found is that while native species should be a strong component of gardens, you don't have to go purely native in order to make a really useful provision for wildlife," says Helen.

However, some cultivated plants have little value for pollinators, including many common bedding plants and anything with heavily doubled flowers (these showy blooms either lack or have inaccessible pollen and nectar), and are probably best used sparingly, especially if you have limited space for plants and you need to get more nectar and pollen-rich bang for your buck. Otherwise, feel free to plant anything you fancy, and you can feel confident you will be creating a thriving garden that supports healthy biodiversity.

# GOOD FOR YOU, GOOD FOR THE PLANET

Growing edible flowers is a wonderful way to connect the dots between gardening, growing your own food, foraging and growing for wildlife. You may not have space for cultivating lots of edibles, but many flowering plants that provide a good source of nectar for pollinators also happen to be delicious for us to eat.

## NASTURTIUM

The peppery seeds taste rather like capers and can be pickled and used in cooking; the flowers are sweet and look pretty in salads; while the leaves add a peppery kick to salads or make a delicious pesto.

## BORAGE

Use the young, tender leaves and flower heads to make a tea infusion with a fresh cucumber flavour. Both leaves and flowers can be enjoyed in salads, but avoid the older, prickly leaves.

## CALENDULA (POT MARIGOLDS)

The edible petals and leaves range from peppery to bitter and can be used in all kinds of dishes. Dry the flower heads and keep for making teas. Calendula has traditionally been used in balms for its soothing and antibacterial qualities.

## CORNFLOWERS

The flowers look pretty in salads, and they pack a flavour punch with their spicy, almost clove-like taste.

## ROSES

The more fragrant and intense in colour, the stronger the flavour. For pollinators, grow traditional single and open-flowered varieties. Pretty as they are, heavily double-flowered tea roses are no use to bees. Use the petals to make rose water or rose syrup that can be used in everything from teas to baking and cocktails; you can also scatter them raw on cakes or salads or crystallize for decorations.

# WILDLIFE-FRIENDLY GARDENING IDEAS

As a general guide, the best wildlife-friendly actions you can take in your garden are as follows.

- Provide food and shelter (including nest boxes, trees and shrubs) for garden birds.

- Let a patch of lawn grow longer throughout the spring and summer (not necessarily the whole lawn).

- Make a pond – even a small one will attract wildlife.

- Plant a flowering tree or a berry-bearing shrub.

- Sow a pot, window box or border with nectar-rich flowering annuals.

- Create habitats – insects love to make homes in log piles, tubes, bug hotels, under plant pots, in piles of leaves and under stones, so leave some less "tidy" spaces for them to hide in.

## COMMUNITY GREEN SPACES

Planting in public spaces is just as important as in our gardens. In Las Vegas, for example, the local water authorities encourage homeowners, developers and businesses to replace "non-functional turf" with more appropriate desert plants, such as succulents and cacti, to reduce the drought-prone city's water consumption and provide richer pickings for pollinators. In the UK, a study revealed that road verges account for 1.2% of the land, and that these spaces support almost half of all the UK's wildflower species.[6] Not surprising given that the UK has lost 97% of its wildflower meadows since the 1930s.

While it's tempting to go out "guerrilla gardening", planting wildflower mixes or using "seed bombs" (which always sound like such a lovely idea) on your neighbourhood verges, the Plantlife charity in the UK, which campaigns for more sustainable management of verges to promote biodiversity, doesn't recommend this approach. Planting generic mixes of wildflower seed does little to conserve wildflowers and can threaten the distinctiveness of natural local species. Instead, mowing less frequently and leaving verges to bloom until autumn (except where they need to be cut back for safety) will give native plants the opportunity to flower and set seed, bringing these important spaces back to life in a natural way and creating habitats for other wildlife. Wherever possible, join with your local community to support reduced mowing in your area – but remember, you have to adjust to a new neighbourhood aesthetic. Getting used to a slightly wilder look in spring will be rewarded with beautiful native flower displays in the summer.

Although technically privately owned, front gardens can be considered a community space because they are at the front of properties and are often on full display for everyone to enjoy. They are also an untapped resource for supporting wildlife and bringing colour and vitality to our neighbourhoods. Increasingly front gardens are being tarmaced or concreted over to provide parking or to reduce maintenance. Research by the London Assembly revealed that in London alone, front garden space that is the equivalent of 5,200 football pitches has been lost to hard landscaping.[7] Not only a loss for wildlife, it also increases the likelihood of flooding as rainwater cannot soak away so easily.

If you are lucky enough to have a front garden, don't be tempted to pave it – plant it abundantly instead. Entrepreneurial growers are even turning front garden spaces into mini allotments, using an otherwise little-used space to grow their own food. It's a wonderful way to get to know your neighbours while you're working on your plot too.

If you do choose to pave a front (or back) garden, try to use permeable materials, such as brick pavers (installed on compacted aggregate) or gravel. From a sustainability perspective, look for recycled materials such as reclaimed bricks or eco-gravel made from waste materials such as bi-product from the ceramics industry.

If your front garden is already hard-landscaped, get creative with climbing plants, containers and shrubs instead. You can even lift the pavers in the centre of your drive, and put low-growing varieties down the middle, proving you can park and plant on the same driveway. There's a plant for every location, however unpromising the conditions seem.

# CHEMICAL IMPACT

Exploring the impact of the over-use of chemical herbicides (which kill weeds) and insecticides (which kill pests) could take up a whole book, but in a nutshell, they damage garden wildlife and potentially pose a threat to human health, especially if used excessively. And the more we use, the more we need to use. It's a particular problem in the US, where blanket spraying of neighbourhoods with pesticides is routine in some areas, a policy supposedly designed to protect people and agriculture that has devastating effects on biodiversity. With some known, and many potentially unknown, repercussions for human health from these chemicals, it seems impossible to justify using them for aesthetic reasons only, such as achieving a weed-free lawn or pest-free roses.

A healthy ecosystem is self-regulating – where there are pests, there's a predator to keep them under control – but chemical pesticides indiscriminately wipe out all wildlife, and eventually the pests also develop an immunity to the chemicals, meaning that a new chemical product must be developed. It's a vicious cycle, but healthy plants generally don't suffer from pest invasions, so if you garden in a more tolerant, natural, wildlife-friendly way, you shouldn't need sprays to remove either weeds or pests.

Also, while you may garden organically, it's worth bearing in mind that your garden centre may not. Research from Sussex University showed that 70% of plants sold at garden centres, supermarkets and DIY stores in the UK contained a cocktail of pesticides, including bee-harming neonicotinoids. A subsequent campaign to remove the most harmful neonicotinoids from garden-centre plants was successful, with many leading garden-centre and horticultural brands promising to stop using them – but there are still many other chemicals used in commercial plant cultivation, not just neonicotinoids. To reduce the impact in your garden, ideally buy from organic garden centres and plant suppliers, grow from seed or plant swap with organic gardener friends.

# A MiNDFUL MoMENT

A simple garden meditation can work wonders. Sit peacefully and take time to see your garden (or any green space such as your local park) through fresh eyes, watching the cycle of nature in action, mindfully tuning into the sights, sounds and aromas of your chosen spot. It's a wonderful reminder of how interdependent all plant and animal species are, and how we are dependent on their survival too.

Focus on imagining the soil being enriched by busy earthworms and micro-organisms breaking down decaying leaf and plant material, locking goodness and carbon into the soil; listen to the hum of pollination; and watch visiting birds plucking insects from the borders. Wildlife encounters are not just for children. If you spot an unusual plant, a different ladybird, an unfamiliar bee or bird, look them up and find out about them. Seeing and discovering something new for yourself is exciting and you never forget these encounters; the names of your discoveries become imprinted in your mind. It's a good way to understand just how many links there are in the biodiversity chain – and how losing even one may eventually lead to the loss of all.

# SIGNPOSTS

For more on:

- Growing herbs, *see* chapter 4
- Health benefits of gardening, *see* chapter 3
- Weeds, wild plants and biodiversity, *see* chapter 12
- Indoor plants, *see* chapter 15
- The importance of trees, *see* chapter 6

# 6

# GROWING HEALTHIER, HAPPIER COMMUNITIES

"A culture is no better than its woods."

WH Auden

---

**THE GOAL:**
**TO PLANT A TREE AND WATCH IT GROW**

**E**VERY TREE HAS A UNIQUE CHARACTER AND SILHOUETTE, growing distinctive foliage, bark, berries and blossom, each adapted to grow in a particular place and to reproduce in its own particular way. Trees grow stories as prolifically as leaves, too, and throughout literature, legend and history these gentle giants have sparked joy, fear and reverence – from the enchanted wood of Enid Blyton's *Magic Faraway Tree* to Shakespeare's powerfully symbolic Forest of Arden in *As You Like It* and the dashing outlaw Robin Hood's fictional oak-tree hideaway. The legendary and quite magnificent Major Oak has thrived in Sherwood Forest not far from where I grew up, for almost a thousand years.

Representing purity, serenity and potency, perhaps longevity is trees' most intriguing superpower, something with which humans, despite all our modern medicines and inventions, cannot compete. Many types outlive us by several generations, some even by millennia, becoming stronger with age as they mark the rings of time in their thickening trunks. General Sherman, the giant sequoia in California's Sequoia National Park is the largest known living single-stem tree on the planet by volume, and it's estimated to be between 2,300 and 2,700 years old. But Sherman is far from being the oldest tree – the current official Guinness record holder is Methuselah in the ancient forests of California's White Mountains, which samples reveal to be over 4,800 years old. Evidence suggests there are other bristlecone pines in the same forest that are older than 5,000 years, but these have not been officially tested and verified.

While trees may be venerable, they are vulnerable too. It only takes minutes for a human with a chainsaw or a bulldozer to fell an ancient tree, bringing a violent end to years of peaceful, productive co-existence. Nowhere is this devastation more significant than in the Amazon. These South American rainforests are the oldest living ecosystems on Earth, with some surviving as they are today since the Cretaceous period, around 66 million years ago. Fossil studies suggest the cataclysmic asteroid collision that triggered the extinction of the dinosaurs at that time also changed rainforests into the modern, much more biodiverse ecosystems that exist today.[1] It's thought the impact and the aftermath reduced plant diversity by up to 45%, but gradually many new varieties emerged, including more flowering plants, which could support a greater range of wildlife, eventually including humans.

It's comforting to know that the forests can recover from such a devastating environmental event – even if it does take a trifling six million years. And that's the thing about deforestation: trees grow incredibly slowly compared to other plants, and it takes longer than a human lifetime to recover a lost ecosystem. Even if the trees do regrow, many dependent species may already have become extinct and the forest will never be quite the same again.

Essential for biodiversity, trees provide, among many other things, habitat for all kinds of species, pollen and nectar for bees and pollinators as well as other food for wildlife and humans, and they bring these benefits regardless of whether they are in a rainforest or an urban neighbourhood. Trees as we recognize them today first evolved around 350 million years ago, and they still shape our landscape as much as modern manmade architecture, providing essential services for which they were not originally designed, yet deliver magnificently – from reducing the temperature in towns and cities by counteracting the "heat island" effect caused by tarmac roads, pavements and buildings, to improving air quality by trapping toxic pollutant particulates in their canopy. At floor level, trees improve soil quality and help prevent erosion and flooding. They make our world beautiful and crucially, they make it habitable, by absorbing vast quantities of carbon from our atmosphere, locking it up in their trunks, leaves, dead wood, leaf mulch, roots and soil.

## WHY RAINFORESTS MATTER

In the time it has taken you to read this sentence, an area of forest at least the size of a football pitch has been cleared in the tropics. Efforts to save tropical forests get a lot of attention, and rightly so, because while estimates vary, research suggests we are losing at least 15 billion trees a year across the world, which is an area around the size of the UK.[2]

It's not a new problem – at the end of the last Ice Age 10,000 years ago, over half of the planet's habitable land was covered by forests, equating to around 6 billion hectares,[3] yet fast forward to today and we have lost a third of our forests with only 4 billion hectares remaining. That may still sound like a lot of forest, but what's concerning is the massive acceleration of deforestation in modern times, as 1 billion hectares were lost gradually between 8,000BC and 1900, while the final billion hectares has gone in just the last hundred years. It's linked with the acceleration in global population growth over the last century; clearing trees to grow crops or graze livestock is the biggest driver of deforestation. Although humans have been doing this for centuries, the scale of the destruction has escalated rapidly in the last century, particularly with the rise in intensive farming, which is why choices we make about how much meat and dairy or products containing palm oil we buy have the potential to make a huge impact on the rate of deforestation.

# THE WOOD-WiDE WEB

While evidence proves that trees create healthier, happier communities for humans, thanks to fascinating ground-breaking research by Dr Suzanne Simard of the University of British Columbia, Canada, we've also learned more in recent years about how social trees are too. We now know they communicate with each other via a vast, complex "wood-wide web" of soil fungi that connects all the vegetation in a woodland or forest, enabling trees to share resources such as sugars and other nutrients and even send out distress or warning signals against insect attacks through their roots. In this way, trees care for ailing neighbours and even feed the stumps of felled trees.

Trees work co-operatively with each other to create a perfectly balanced microclimate in which they can store water, regulate extremes of temperatures and generate humidity, and this is partly why forest trees in particular can live to such a ripe old age. The question is – if trees understand the benefits of working co-operatively to maintain a healthy environment, surely we can too?

Nearly all (95%) of this deforestation is happening in the tropics, much of it driven by demand for products such as beef, vegetable oil, cocoa, coffee and paper from the world's richest countries. It's not just the Amazon rainforests under threat, of course, and the WWF has identified several areas at risk of catastrophic forest loss, including the Atlantic Forest/Gran Chaco, spanning Paraguay, Brazil and Argentina, along with Borneo, the Congo Basin, Eastern Africa, Eastern Australia and the Greater Mekong.[4]

Tropical forests in particular are home to some of the richest and most diverse ecosystems on the planet. Over half of the world's species reside in tropical forests[5] and these ecosystems are rich in unique wildlife that is not found anywhere else in the world. Habitat loss is the leading cause of global biodiversity loss, and these ecosystems will never be the same again, even if they are reforested.

But the risks from deforestation go further. All trees absorb and store carbon dioxide. When forests are cleared and the soil ploughed for agriculture this carbon is released, along with other greenhouse gases, into the atmosphere. Although there are many "carbon sinks" in a variety of terrestrial and aquatic ecosystems – the ocean is the largest carbon sink on the planet, and other types of ecosystems such as the mangrove swamps of Indonesia are also important – tropical and subtropical forests are saturated in sequestered carbon. The Amazon rainforests alone store 90–140 billion tonnes,[6] which is why forest loss and damage is the cause of around 10% of global warming.

The bottom line is: if we don't fight deforestation in the tropics, we cannot effectively fight climate change. It's like trying to fill a bath with no plug.

# WHAT'S THE LiNK BETWEEN PALM OiL AND DEFORESTATiON?

Palm oil is one of the more ethically problematic plant crops, and it's found in all kinds of household products from shampoo to cookies. It's incredibly hard to avoid, even if you are an eco-conscious shopper, as up to 50% of products in the average UK supermarket contain palm oil.[7] Apparently, on average we each consume globally around 8kg (17½lb) of the stuff each year, which is a rather unappetizing thought. And if you buy meat and dairy products, chances are the animals have been given feed containing palm oil too.

As consumers and then manufacturers turned away from using saturated fats and trans fats found in partially hydrogenated oils because of the links with heart disease, virtually all the trans fats in processed foods were substituted with palm oil as a healthier alternative. However, as demand for palm oil has grown and plantations have spread, increasingly vast areas of carbon-sequestering rainforests rich in biodiversity continue to be cleared, while palm plantations can't support native wildlife. Numbers of unique species are already at risk; populations of pygmy elephants, Sumatran tigers, three species of orangutans and Sumatran rhino are all diminishing rapidly because of this habitat loss.[8]

Initially, the solution seemed to be a boycott. But the economy of countries such as Malaysia and Indonesia are heavily dependent on palm oil exports, and many communities would be at great risk of poverty without this industry.

Palms are uniquely high-yielding, which means alternative oils may have even worse environmental consequences – crops like rapeseed (canola) oil, for example, would need up to nine times more land to produce the same volume of oil.

Palm oil is a naturally sustainable crop when it's grown in the right way and not in wildly escalating volumes. Most leading conservation organizations, including the WWF, support sustainable palm oil as a more realistic option, one that is positive for people and planet. It's not a perfect solution, but it is a real-world one.

Sustainable palm oil is grown without deforestation and must be produced in a way that reduces its impact on biodiversity and supports human rights. The Round Table on Palm Oil (RSPO) sets best practices for the industry, although while these standards are generally considered to be the most robust of those available, many environmentalists believe they are far from perfect.[9]

As consumers, we also have a part to play here. Our global appetite for animal products and processed foods is directly leading to deforestation and endangering irreplaceable species such as orangutans in the process. To help change happen, look for brands and products that contain sustainable palm oil. The WWF produces a useful annual Palm Oil Buyers Scorecard,[10] and Chester Zoo in the UK provides lots of great resources at chesterzoo.org.[11]

# 3 WAYS TO PLANT TREES — NO SPADE REQUIRED

It's easy to feel powerless to do anything, as most of us have no direct control over the activities of governments, logging companies, cattle ranchers or palm oil producers in at-risk regions. But we can support tree-planting schemes in a small way from the comfort of our sofa.

## 1 THERE'S AN APP FOR THAT

A plethora of new tree-planting apps now enable you to plant trees without breaking a sweat. Treekly is one such example (treekly.org), which cleverly incentivizes people to do more daily steps to earn free trees, which Treekly plants in Madagascar as part of an ambitious plan to both combat sedentary lifestyles and plant millions of trees. With any kind of offsetting scheme, look for transparency about where trees are planted and ensure they offer regular reporting on progress for accountability.

## 2 DON'T GOOGLE IT

Instead of using Google on autopilot, switch to the green search engine Ecosia, which generates income from search ads and uses the money to plant trees in places such as Brazil, Indonesia and Burkino Faso. Ecosia says it removes 1kg (2lb 4oz) of $CO_2$ for every internet search, plus their servers run on renewable energy. To make it second nature to use Ecosia, set it as your default search engine (full instructions are on Ecosia's website) or download the app to your phone.

## 3 GOING ON A SHOPPING "TREE"

Many companies now claim to plant a tree when you buy goods or services from them. Do be a savvy consumer though, as the growth of tree-planting schemes means it's even easier for companies to "greenwash" their products, services and operations – for example, by partnering with a tree-planting organization (which may be entirely reputable) to plant a tree for every product sold, while continuing to be wasteful, polluting or exploitative of people and planet in other respects.

# DOES CARBON OFFSETTiNG WORK?

Offsetting works by allowing people to invest money in schemes that plant trees, reduce deforestation or develop renewable sources of energy, so while you can't cancel out the $CO_2$ already generated by your flight, you can help reduce total global emissions by funding a carbon-positive project. However, offsetting can't be seen as a free pass to carry on as normal, it's just one tool you can use in partnership with changing habits and reducing your overall carbon footprint.

However, some experts are not convinced that the science behind offsetting stacks up. Mike Berners-Lee, author of *How Bad Are Bananas,* criticizes cheap schemes that allow people to offset their jet-setting habits for as little as £3 per tonne of $CO^2e$. "All such cheap 'offset' options turn out to be fatally flawed and/or fundamentally limited in scope," he says. "They are often about things like solar power or tree planting that we need anyway to reach carbon zero – and we can't just use them to counterbalance our emissions."[12]

If you would like to offset, look for a scheme that is independently accredited and openly shares data on its impacts from previous years. Tree planting schemes need to be planting the right trees in the right places and should be providing employment opportunities for – and not displacing – indigenous communities in the process.

It's also worth remembering that it takes trees a long time to grow and planting swathes of saplings cannot compensate for the loss of existing ancient forests, which have enormous carbon sequestering capacity and richer biodiversity compared to new woodland. For this reason, it's better to

invest in conservation rather than new tree planting –
Sir David Attenborough is a patron of worldlandtrust.org
and this organization focuses on protecting existing forest
and ecosystems.

## GOOD FOR YOU, GOOD FOR THE PLANET

Using apps and tree planting schemes is great up to a point, but there's
nothing like getting your own hands dirty. It may seem like a small thing but
planting even one tree in your garden does help, on a neighbourhood level
and beyond. There's such a simple joy in planting a sapling with your own
hands and watching it grow. You don't have to be much of a gardener to do
it, but if you choose the right tree you'll be planting a legacy that could last
a century or even more.

If you like your garden to be a mindful space, research has shown that
birdsong and wind rustling in the trees are two of the most relaxing sounds
in nature[13] – and trees will bring both sounds into your garden.

But what type of tree should you grow? Tree planting charities, gardening
organizations and garden centres often produce lists of the best species to
grow in your area, but the best choice really comes down to the eventual
size and spread of the tree, the planting location, growing conditions and
personal preferences. If you like the idea of harvesting something edible every
year, choose a fruit tree; or if you live near a busy road, consider something
with hairy, waxy or rough leaves, such as hawthorn, red cedar or cotoneaster,
which are known to be particularly effective at trapping tiny airborne
particulate pollutants. It's estimated that trees and other plants remove
around 1.3 billion kg of health-harming air pollutants in the UK every year.[14]

Even a very small garden can accommodate a tree and there are many
types of naturally neat flowering varieties that will fit nicely into a smaller
space. You could also opt for a container tree or shrub for a courtyard or

balcony. Varieties such as Japanese maples, dwarf conifers, and bay, olive, holly, restricted crab apple and apple trees (grown on a semi-dwarfing rootstock) will all thrive in a heavy, stable container, although potted trees will need more maintenance with watering and feeding, and some varieties will need protecting from frosts.

"All types of trees have benefits, so plant something you like and that will not need pruning when it reaches full size," advises chartered arboriculturalist Russell Horsey. "Not only does this mean less maintenance, but some trees like birch don't like it, and eventually pruning may kill them. So don't plant a mighty oak if there's only space for a small apple tree."

Buying locally grown saplings also reduces the growing problem of imported tree-harming pests and diseases, but while some people argue we should stick to growing native species, Russell believes this isn't always the most important consideration. "As our climate changes, non-native species may prove to be more resilient and have a better chance of survival – and help other species that depend on them survive too. So, just choose a tree you love and both you and future generations will enjoy the benefits."

# HOW TO PLANT A TREE

Once you've chosen your tree species, here's your step-by-step guide to successful planting. Peak tree-planting season is in the autumn (fall) to early spring when the trees are dormant and less likely to be damaged. It's a lovely project to bring joy to your garden in the winter months.

- Choose the best location for your sapling, taking into consideration the eventual size and spread of the fully grown tree and its potential impact on buildings, paths and other trees.

- Remove the tree from its pot and stand it in a bucket of water to thoroughly soak the root ball before planting.

- Dig a pit for your tree, which should be the same depth as the root ball and at least three times the width.

- Using your fingers, loosen the root ball. This encourages the roots to grow into the surrounding soil.

- Place the tree in the pit. The point where the root ball meets the trunk should be level with the soil surface – you can use a plank of wood to check, if necessary.

- Fill the pit with soil around the root ball, firming it down to avoid leaving any air pockets. Ensure your tree isn't wonky – ideally ask someone to hold it straight while you fill the hole.

- Depending on where your tree is located, you may want to consider adding a tree guard to protect it against hungry wildlife, especially deer.

- Water the tree base thoroughly and then add a layer of mulch such as bark chippings, but don't mulch right up to the tree stem, leave a bit of clear space all around.

- If it's a tall, top-heavy tree you may need to add a stake at a 45-degree angle to keep it secure.

- Your new tree will benefit from regular watering throughout the first 2–3 years while the roots become established, especially during hot, dry spells.

# GROWING GREENER COMMUNITIES

Next time you walk through your neighbourhood, take a moment to notice how many trees you pass by – I'm willing to bet there are more trees in your vicinity than you expected to count. Many of us walk past numerous trees every day, taking their presence for granted. But this lovely leafiness is vanishing fast, as over the last 50 years, trees have been disappearing from our neighbourhoods at a worrying rate.

Part of the problem is a legacy of poorly planned planting, which means that over time trees planted by previous generations become too large or unsuitable for their location. When these older trees die, become diseased or start to create problems such as uprooting pavements, it's often easier for cash-strapped local authorities to simply remove the trees, and they are rarely replaced.

While the gradual disappearance of trees from urban areas doesn't get the publicity that deforestation in the Amazon does, the environmental impact can still be significant, especially when no one is keeping count of the losses. When beautiful old trees are felled, it quite rightly arouses strong emotions in the local community, particularly when there's no good reason for their removal. The scandal of widespread and unnecessary urban tree felling in Sheffield, UK, in 2017 – over 5,000 trees – caused an outcry, locally, nationally and even internationally, and the Sheffield Street Tree Partnership was formed to protect the remaining trees. But trees are disappearing from all of our towns and cities and there's not always a big splash in the media about it.

Sarah Shorley, of the Urban Tree Team at the Woodland Trust charity, says: "To me it seems crazy that in the UK not all local councils have a tree policy to set out a clear plan for how they manage, protect and plant trees in their area," she says. "There's an increasing recognition that urban forestry is about people and creating healthier environments for us to live in. Sometimes I look at all the concrete in our towns and cities and just feel so frustrated about what we've done to this planet. It's going to take an incredible amount of work to redress the balance."

Sadly, it seems that even protecting trees in our neighbourhoods often seems to come down to budget, or lack of it, and whether trees are "earning their keep" in some way, by providing vital services such as urban cooling or reducing pollution.

"Everything seems to revolve around economy and quantifying the benefits trees can bring financially," agrees Sarah. "But I absolutely believe trees should be valued just for being trees, for the beauty they bring to our spaces. They make our environment look better and we feel better when we look at them. The health and wellbeing benefits are palpable."

Community action group Save Our Street Trees was founded by local resident Alice Whitehead in Northampton, UK, with a mission to restore lost street trees to the town. "Internationally, groups like Save Our Street Trees are working on projects to replace these trees," she says. "When they go, we lose a multitude of benefits. Not just for wildlife – lots of studies show they have huge impact on social cohesion and create closer, safer communities. Research shows that where there are more trees there is less litter, less antisocial behaviour and less crime."

The story is similar in the USA too, where a study revealed that US cities are losing 29 million trees every year. In Baltimore, for example, there is considerably more greenery in affluent areas, an imbalance that the Baltimore Tree Trust is trying to address with an equitably distributed tree-planting programme to provide much-needed canopy in a city that experiences swelteringly hot summers.[15] A comment from Justin Bowers, COO of the Baltimore Tree Trust, captures just how important trees are to the infrastructure of our built environment: "People are waking up to the idea that a healthy network of trees and green spaces is as vital to the livability of cities as other public utilities, like roads and sewers."[16]

Trees don't just improve social deprivation or provide benefits for physical health, they play an important role in supporting mental wellbeing, which is why Alice believes that while parks and woodlands are important, trees should be woven into the fabric of our neighbourhoods. "The closer the trees are to people's houses, the more benefits they bring," she says. "It's great to have trees in parks and urban woodland areas, but it's vital to have trees on streets not just in enclaves. It's especially important in built-up areas where people have fewer gardens or there are lots of apartment blocks. Research suggests that just being able to see a view of nature from a window can have a positive impact on mental health as much as being in a park full of trees."

## TREES, TREES EVERYWHERE

While making tree planting – and a plan and budget for maintaining them – mandatory in all urban planning decisions for the future would undoubtedly help to create healthier, happier neighbourhoods, can tree planting in every available space we can find really help save the planet too? It's a hot topic right now, as research suggesting that planting millions of trees and restoring woodlands could be the simplest and most low-tech solution to climate change has captured the public imagination and empowered people to start digging for victory.

Working in conjunction with efforts to reduce emissions from industry, agriculture and transport, it's thought that planting 1.2 trillion trees globally could remove a decade's worth of human-activity-generated carbon emissions from the atmosphere over the next 50–100 years.[17]

As an example, with just less than a quarter of the UK's land area covered by trees (compared to the EU average of 37%), cover would ideally need to increase from 13 to at least 19%, adding 1.5 million hectares (3.7 million acres) of woodland – but the experts say there is plenty of space to achieve this through a range of approaches including agroforestry. Although it's vitally important to protect ancient woodland, a young wood with mixed native species can still lock up over 400 tonnes of carbon per hectare, while agroforestry, which combines tree planting with agricultural and pastureland, can have even wider benefits such as more sustainable food production, improved soil quality and increased biodiversity.

There are a lot of big numbers being thrown around when it comes to tree planting schemes. Back in 1990 in Chicago, Mayor Richard Daley announced an ambitious programme to plant half a million trees, making him something of an eco-pioneer at the time, and the UK is catching up to the idea. It seems to make perfect sense: climate change is caused by rising carbon emissions – trees sequester carbon – so let's plant more trees. Glasgow, for example, has announced plans to plant 18 million trees over the next decade, connecting existing swathes of broadleaved woodland, creating important wildlife corridors. The project is part of the Clyde Climate Forest, part of the city's commitment to reaching net zero carbon emissions.

However, some schemes are less well thought through, and the numbers don't always add up. "Young trees, around 1–2 years old and 40cm (16in) tall, could be planted into woodland, but you probably have to plant at least 3,000 to eventually get 100 mature trees," says Russell. "That's why the numbers game is a little bit of a myth – you can say you're planting a million trees, but in a hundred years' time how many will still be there? Only a very small percentage will make it to maturity. This is why mapping suitable spaces to plant trees where they are most likely to grow successfully is so important. It's far better to plant fewer trees but in the right places."

# HOW TO SET UP A COMMUNITY TREE-PLANTING PROJECT

1.  If you have one in your area, join an existing group and support your community to plant trees. www.saveour-streettrees.org has a useful list of international groups.

2.  If there is no group, set up your own. You'll need to consider aspects such as opening a bank account, creating a management committee, connecting with experienced arboriculturalists or tree charities and growing an engaged community through a website, social media, word of mouth and local events to keep the momentum going. It's worth connecting with other community groups for support and advice too.

3.  Tempting as it may be to try "guerilla" tree planting, you need considerable expertise to do this well. Trees won't grow properly if the conditions are not right and if they are not maintained in the early years. Plus, if you plant on private or local authority land without permission, your trees may be removed.

4.  You may feel that not enough is being done, but it's very important to work positively and constructively with local authorities, residents, landowners, developers, contractors and other involved parties to achieve your goals. Communication with all stakeholders is key to successful tree-planting schemes.

5.  Location, location, location is everything – identify where you are going to plant trees before you order a tree pack. Talk to local landowners, farmers, schools, housing associations, developers and the local authority to find suitable locations and get all the necessary permissions in place.

6.  Consult an expert to decide which species and quantity of trees will thrive best in your available location, factoring in the eventual height and spread of the species you choose.

7.  Order your trees and invite your community to help with planting – throwing a bit of a party encourages people to join in the fun.

# SIGNPOSTS

For more on:

❀ Deforestation, agriculture, and food choices, *see* chapters 2, 5 and 10

❀ Health and wellbeing benefits of trees, *see* chapters 1 and 6

❀ Foraging for wild foods, *see* chapter 12

❀ Plants and air quality, *see* chapter 15

❀ Garden biodiversity, *see* chapter 5

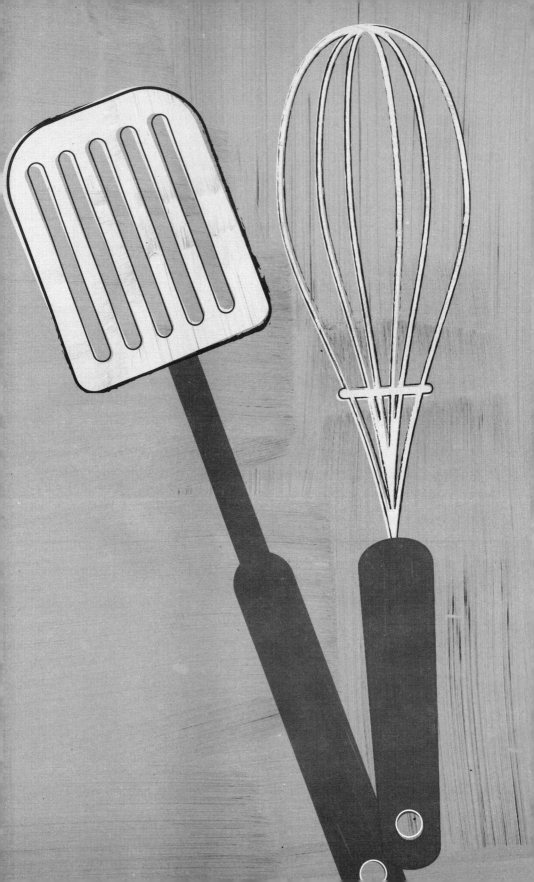

# COOK

Living plantfully is all about celebrating the power of plants and putting them at the heart and centre of your life, and particularly on your plate. Being mindful of where food comes from and how it is produced; eating more seasonal, local ingredients; and aiming to use every leaf, peel and root you possibly can once it reaches your kitchen are all so important because our food is such a precious resource. Reducing animal products creates space to be adventurous with plant ingredients, which not only makes your diet more exciting, nourishing and full of diverse flavours, it's also a more sustainable and kinder way of eating that does less harm to people, planet and animals. This is a life-enhancing, label-free way of eating that will make you happier and healthier.

# 7

# PLANT POSITIVITY

"If you want to win more people over to the veg camp, there is no worse way to go about it than demand we go cold turkey."

Yotam Ottolenghi, *Flavour*

**THE GOAL:**
**TO FIND CREATIVE WAYS TO GET MORE PLANTS ON YOUR PLATE**

**P**AST EXPERIENCES WITH POORLY COOKED VEGGIES CAN LINGER in the memory like the aroma of over-boiled cabbage in a school dinner hall. As someone who grew up eating broccoli that was cooked ferociously for at least 20 minutes (sorry Mum), I understand why people may well feel a little prejudiced against greens later in life. But if I can forgive broccoli and enjoy it now – more appetisingly cooked and presented, of course – anyone can.

Plants don't just keep us healthy; when prepared and cooked in the right way, they are so full of flavour too. There's definitely more to tempt the tastebuds in a morsel of miso-roasted aubergine (eggplant) than a dull slice of grilled chicken, while a rainbow of vibrant vegetables surely looks more appetizing on the plate than the dull beige-brownness of meat. In fact, while many mammals rely mostly on their sense of smell to find and appreciate food, humans have evolved a sophisticated ability to detect and respond more to colour, a skill that enables us to find good things to eat in nature, such as ripe fruits – so the science backs up the idea that we eat with our eyes first.

Living plantfully is a more abundant, colourful way of eating. It's about filling your plate with delicious, nourishing foods and a much greater variety of vibrant flavours, providing the nutrients you need to maintain a healthy weight, feel more energized and enjoy other benefits such as glowing skin and glossy hair. By nurturing a better balance in your diet, you'll create a happier, healthier, more harmonious you.

Which is why, instead of beginning this journey by talking about reducing or replacing meat, we'll start by getting more creative with how we use plants in the kitchen. It's time to knock meat off its pedestal and let plants step into the limelight as the stars of the show.

We need a change of mindset to prepare for a future of eating predominantly plants. Not just individually but culturally, and on a global scale. Around 90% of the world's population are meat eaters and the global rate of consumption is rising – the world eats a whopping 340 million tonnes of it every year.[1] It's not sustainable for our health, the planet or for animal welfare to keep eating this volume of meat. As Professor Sir

Charles Godfray, population biologist and co-director of the LEAP project (Livestock, Environment and People) at the University of Oxford, says: "It's just not possible to produce enough meat for everyone to eat the way people do in wealthier countries – we need a difficult but urgent discussion on the amount of meat we consume."

At the very least, meat needs to step back from the starring role and join the supporting cast. Breaking the habit of making meat the centrepiece of every meal shouldn't be difficult if we put our minds to it, because satisfying and nutritious dishes can be based around vegetables, fruits, pulses, grains, nuts, seeds, herbs and spices alone – and nothing is "missing". There are already 2 billion people on the planet eating a meat-free diet – meat is not essential for survival.

It may be helpful to try to think differently about what a "proper" meal should look like on the plate. Traditionally, many of us have grown up in a culture where there is usually a meat or fish-based centrepiece, while many dishes we eat regularly are defined by the "main ingredient", such as a chicken curry, even if it's packed with other ingredients such as mushrooms and kale too. Perhaps we could take inspiration from cultures where mezze or tapas-style eating is common, where a collection of dishes are presented with equal importance and everyone digs in and enjoys a little of each, which is a wonderful way to introduce a wide variety of ingredients and flavours in one meal. Or to start planning meals around your plant foods first to make them the centrepiece, with meat and dairy products added as sides for those in the family who still eat them.

Hundreds of types of plant ingredients can be combined in thousands of ways to make delicious and nutritious meals, and you only have to compare this infinite variety to the limited range of meat and fish products most people consume regularly to see the possibilities. Food writers are producing incredibly exciting meat- and dairy-free recipes now, so there's endless inspiration out there.

Regardless of whether you consider yourself to be vegan, veggie, flexitarian or carnivore, at least half of your plate at every meal should be filled with vegetables and fruit anyway. Getting the balance right is so important to help you look and feel your best. In the USA and UK, average daily intake of fruit and veg falls far short of the recommended minimum.[2] In many wealthier countries, the wide availability of cheap, ultra-processed foods means the balance between wholefoods and processed is completely out of kilter. Over half of the average UK diet is made from ultra-processed foods,[3] and it's a similar story in the USA.

When it comes to good health, balance is everything. So don't start by thinking in extremes: "I have to give up all meat" or "I have to go vegan tomorrow". First, focus on something simple and achievable – upping your intake of minimally processed plant foods. Writing a food diary will help you get a clearer picture of the balance of your current diet and give you something to aim for, such as filling at least half your plate with vegetables at every meal. Remember, you are doing this for you – so feel free to go at your own pace.

# GET YOUR 30-A-WEEK

We could all benefit from switching up our fruit and veg repertoire. Do you ever buy gooseberries, apricots, fennel or chicory (endive)? Do you eat the same old apple or banana every day? Recent research by the British Nutrition Foundation revealed that in the UK half of people's veg intake is focused on just four types: peas, tomatoes, onions and carrots, which sounds very dull. Eating an abundance of plants is key to providing all the fibre, vitamins, minerals and phytonutrients we need for optimum health, and all the flavours we need to really enjoy our food. People in the UK are very familiar with the "five-a-day" concept that's been ingrained in public health advice for almost 20 years, but a recent Imperial College London project analysed 95 international studies on fruit and veg intake and concluded that if people ate ten 80g (3oz) portions a day, 7.8 million premature deaths every year could be prevented worldwide.[4]

Whatever the magic number of daily fruit and veg may be, too many people are not eating even close to the minimum recommendation, so anything we can do to get closer to seven to ten portions a day will have a huge impact on our health. Research from the American Gut Project and the British Gut

Project, which tested microbiome samples from over 11,000 people, led to a "30-a-week" campaign. The results of DNA tests to identify strains of microbes in the samples revealed that people eating 30 or more different plant foods a week had the most diverse gut bacteria and fewer antibiotic resistance genes in their gut microbiomes than people who ate 10 or fewer plants.[5] Different good gut microbes feast on different types of dietary fibres, so for healthy bacterial diversity you need diet diversity.

Keeping that idea of "30 a week" in mind is a good way to focus on improving variety in your diet – why not keep a list on the fridge door each week and every time you eat a portion of plant foods, add it to the list? Challenge the whole family to join in too. Before you panic that you can't even name 30 different types of fruits and vegetables, for this exercise plant foods also include seeds, nuts, wholegrains, beans, pulses, herbs and spices. A portion is usually considered to be 80g (3oz), or 30g (1oz) for nuts and seeds, but the quality and diversity of the food is more important than exact quantities.

As a guide, keep the following tips in mind when you're buying plant foods:

- Choose minimally processed wholefoods wherever possible, such as brown rice and wholegrain bread, and use the skins and leaves of fruit and vegetables.

- Convenience options such as pre-chopped veg are fine occasionally – and certainly better than less healthy alternatives – but for maximum nutrient content try to buy whole fruit and veg and prep it yourself as much as possible. It will save you money too.

- Buy a wide range of colours and varieties of plant foods, and vary them each week to get your 30 ticked off.

- Enjoy a balance of raw and cooked foods in your diet, as some nutrients are more available when food is raw or cooked. For example, the antioxidant lycopene is more abundant in cooked tomatoes, while water-soluble vitamin C is often damaged by heat or leaches into cooking water.

- Prioritize local, seasonal produce as much as you can, as this usually means it has better flavour, is more nutritious and has a lower carbon footprint too.

- Buy the best quality you can afford, including Fairtrade, organic or regeneratively farmed produce, if it's within your budget.

- Use fruit and veg while they are as fresh as possible – don't let them linger in the fridge too long. Frozen fruit and veg can be a great standby and may be more beneficial than fresh food left to deplete its nutrients in the fridge for a week.

# 5 TRICKS TO GET YOUR 30 A WEEK

For a short and sweet way to maximize the number of plant varieties in every meal, every time you're preparing food, keep these five steps in mind:

1. **Change** up your grain – leave the pasta and rice in the cupboard and switch to something different, such as freekeh, pearl barley or buckwheat.

2. **Pack** in a pulse – add something from the pea, bean and lentil family, which could be foods such as tofu, edamame beans, hummus, lentils or peas.

3. **Chop** one more vegetable or fruit – there's always space on the plate for one more veg variety – or finish your meal with a piece of fruit.

4. **Add** a flavour bomb – a handful of fresh herbs or a scattering of spices brings powerful flavour and antioxidants to your dish.

5. **Finish** with a sprinkle of something – seeds and nuts (and seed and nut butters) are a nutritious finishing touch for every dish.

# 12 EASY WAYS TO PACK IN MORE VEG

When you start focusing on upping your intake of plant foods, you'll soon start to see every meal and snack as an opportunity to squeeze in even more greens – and reds, yellows and purples. Get creative with sweet recipes too – you can add grated carrot to porridge, beans to brownies and courgette (zucchini) to muffins. Get in the habit of always topping your breakfast with fruit, and every time you make a savoury recipe, add one extra vegetable that isn't listed in the ingredients.

In the spirit of improving the variety of the plants you eat, here are some easy ways you can start eating a wider range of plant foods – all without making major changes to your diet.

## 1 START SMALL

Trying to do too much at once can be overwhelming, so start by making a change for one meal of the day. Try a plant-based milk for breakfast and adding fruit as a topping or purée. Or make all packed lunches meat-free for work and school.

## 2 CHOOSE A NEW "VEG OF THE WEEK"

Pick a new-to-you or rarely-used vegetable each week. If you never buy more unusual varieties such as fennel or kohlrabi, research recipes to use them in. Get the whole family involved in choosing the "veg of the week".

## 3 COOK IT DIFFERENTLY

I can't emphasize enough that the cooking method is terribly important for getting the best out of veggies, so if you always boil or steam vegetables, try different ways to prepare them such as roasting or stir frying, and see how it changes the flavour and texture. For example, boiled or even steamed cauliflower can go soggy in the blink of an eye, and it leaves that lingering sulphurous aroma in the house. But eaten raw or roasted, cauliflower tastes like a completely different vegetable.

## 4 STOCK UP ON FROZEN OPTIONS

When you start to use more vegetables, you'll notice you're doing a lot more peeling and chopping. We can be a bit snobby about frozen veg, but they are often just as nutritious, especially if your "fresh" veg has been languishing in your fridge for days. In some cases, the nutrient content can be higher in frozen than fresh – for example, frozen blueberries have more vitamin C Frozen options are often best for when you want to eat produce that is out of season and in dishes where the texture doesn't matter so much – frozen summer berries are perfect for adding to smoothies or stirring into porridge. Harder-to-prep veg such as butternut squash cubes can make whizzing up a soup, curry or a stew so much easier. Some of the best frozen veg to have on standby are cauliflower rice, spinach (which spoils quickly when fresh) for adding straight to cooked dishes, green beans, broccoli (roast from frozen rather than boil or defrost, or use for pesto), frozen (bell) peppers for stir fries, sweetcorn, shelled edamame and peas.

## 5 COOK FROM SCRATCH

This is a big change, and it can be hard if you rely a lot on readymade products. Don't try to do everything at once – start with one product you normally buy readymade and make it from scratch to establish a new habit. Then move onto something else. This could be a soup for your weekday lunches or hummus, pesto or pasta sauce, if you normally buy readymade varieties. Making your own means you can experiment using different ingredients and you can control the oil, sugar and salt levels too. Batch cooking and freezing extra portions of meals or components such as sauces whenever possible will save time and effort another day.

## 6 GO AGAINST THE GRAIN

If you always use "mainstream" grains such as rice and couscous, try adding in some alternative grains. Quinoa is high in protein and offers a complete range of amino acids, while freekeh, farro and bulgur are higher in fibre than traditional wheat grains. Spelt and pearl barley are great alternatives to white arborio rice for risotto, while adding wild rice to a salad or pilaf will boost the plant-based protein. Try buckwheat flour for pancakes instead of white flour, while readymade chickpea- (gram-), lentil- or edamame-flour pasta or noodles are higher in protein.

## 7 SEASON'S EATINGS

Try to start eating in harmony with the seasons. Not only does this reduce food miles, it can also save you money because you are buying locally grown produce at its most naturally abundant time, when costs are lower for suppliers. Reducing travel time and distance from field to plate also ensures produce is at its peak of flavour and goodness. There are lots of resources online to find out what's in season where you live.

## 8 SIGN UP FOR A VEG BOX

This is a great idea, especially if it's organic produce. Not only will you be getting good quality, predominantly locally-grown produce and cutting down on food miles, you'll also be reducing plastic packaging waste. Because the box contents change with the seasons and are often a surprise, you have to be a little adventurous with your cooking to use things up, and many box schemes provide recipe ideas too. Also, you'll naturally learn to eat more seasonally this way – and start to look forward to certain fruit and veg becoming available throughout the year. National box delivery companies can be fantastic (and often offer far more than just veg), but do check if you have any local schemes, as smaller independent veg box suppliers can be very good value.

## 9 SWAP A SNACK

This is a fun one. For most of us, snacks probably won't be meat-based anyway, but they may well be processed foods such as granola bars or crisps. Challenge yourself to change snacks to more natural, wholefood, plant-based options, from oven-roasted vegetable "crisps" to spice-roasted nuts, homemade energy balls, crispy chickpeas (garbanzo beans), dried fruit slices or veg-and-bean-based dips with crudités.

## 10 PACK IN THE FLAVOUR

Cooked the right way, vegetables have amazing natural flavours, but sometimes people miss the "umami" savoury taste that foods such as meat bring to a dish. Try cooking with ingredients that have a unique depth of flavour, such as miso, dried porcini mushrooms, smoked paprika, soya sauce or tamari, pomegranate molasses, nutritional yeast flakes, chipotle or chilli paste, harissa, garlic, fresh and dried herbs and spices. A great way to bring simply cooked veggies to life and make them more interesting for those who are less keen is to add a touch of sparkle in the form of a dip, drizzle or topping. This could be a spoonful of homemade pesto, a squeeze of lemon, a pinch of garlic or chilli salt, a sprinkle of toasted or spice-roasted seeds or nuts, a drizzle of a flavoursome oil such as sesame or walnut, a scattering of fresh herbs or a dash of something spicy like chilli jam or sriracha sauce. However, try to avoid sugary processed sauces such as ketchup, or adding table salt.

## 11 ENHANCE WITH PLANTS

Think about the dishes you make regularly and how you could pack more veg into existing favourites – this way, the family might be more willing to accept them. If they love cottage pie, you could halve the mince (ground meat), swap in some brown lentils, and add some more finely chopped vegetables, which will melt into the rich sauce, adding nutrients but without changing the flavour too much. Or in a chicken curry, reduce the chicken and add chickpeas (garbanzo beans) and spinach instead, then serve with cauliflower rice or 50/50 rice and cauliflower. Introducing the plant alternatives alongside meat is a gentler transition, and helps the family gradually get used to some new flavours and textures. For dishes you make regularly, change the veg you normally use – so next time you make mash, try using sweet potato, or a mix of potato and celeriac (celery root) or even butterbean mash.

## 12 DON'T FORGET TEXTURE

Often, it's the satisfying mouthfeel of meat that people miss the most, so think about how to incorporate "meaty" textures into your cooking. Mushrooms are great for this – especially large chunky varieties such as king oysters and portobello, but grilled aubergine (eggplant), jackfruit (which can be used to recreate dishes such as hoisin duck and pulled pork), tofu, tempeh or seitan also work well. Nuts and seeds are another way to add a delicious and nutritious crunchy texture to vegetable dishes.

# THE DiRTY DOZEN

When it comes to fruit and veg, upgrading to organic is usually worth paying for. Organic is not the perfect solution but it is a less intensive, more natural agricultural system that is gentler on the environment and produces food with lower levels of contamination by chemicals such as fertilizers and pesticides, so it's a big step in the right direction. If you can't afford to buy all organic, then focus on upgrading the "dirty dozen", the top 12 most contaminated non-organic fruit and veg. This list is issued every year by the Environmental Working Group, although the 12 culprits don't tend to vary much, and if you eat any of the produce on this list regularly, it's worth trying to find organic if possible.

- Strawberries
- Spinach
- Kale/collard and mustard greens
- Nectarines
- Apples
- Grapes
- Cherries
- Peaches
- Pears
- Bell and hot peppers
- Celery
- Tomatoes

# THE MISSING MACRONUTRIENT

You've undoubtedly heard a lot about gut health lately – who knew we'd all suddenly become so interested in the contents of our colons? But it's important to be aware of our microbiome, because there's a fascinating battle between "good" and "bad" bacteria going on in there that sounds a little like the plotline of a superhero movie.

Our microbiome is an internal ecosystem of 40 trillion bacteria found in the gut, the balance of which changes continually throughout our lives, depending on factors such as diet and lifestyle. Evidence suggests that the microbiome and brain are in constant communication, and that the concept of having "a gut feeling" may actually be backed up by science.

In fact, we now know that the microbiome has a much bigger and more important job than previously thought, as all these bacteria have a complex, interdependent role to play in almost every system and function of the body, from boosting immunity to helping prevent chronic illnesses, including cancer. It's an intriguing yet relatively new area of research and exciting discoveries are being made all the time. However, what we do know is that limiting dairy, red and processed meats and refined sugar has been shown to improve gut health, as does eating nutrient- and fibre-rich foods such as vegetables, wholegrains, nuts and seeds.

The link between a plant-centred diet and a healthy gut microbiome is fibre. In the UK, government guidelines say we should be eating at least 30g (1oz) fibre every day to keep our digestive system working well, but most people are only averaging 18g (under ¾oz).[6]

"Our good gut bacteria exclusively eat fibre," explains Lisa Simon, a dietitian focusing on gut health. "So, if you want more anti-inflammatory bacteria to flourish, this means eating more plant-based foods. There is no fibre in animal products whatsoever, so if you eat a typical Western diet high in meat and dairy products that is also high in fat and sugar, then you are creating the perfect environment for the "bad" inflammatory bacteria to thrive, as this is what sustains them. By contrast, if you eat lots of plant foods, the good bacteria will break those down into short-chain fatty acids, which are beneficial for pretty much everything in your body, including brain function. The more anti-inflammatory bacteria you have, the better it is for your health."

So, we know a happy gut is fuelled by lots of fibre, but what it really doesn't like is ultra-processed junk foods. "These foods are full of ingredients the gut doesn't want or need," says Lisa. "They are high in saturated fat, salt and sugar, plus they contain artificial sweeteners, additives, preservatives and other chemicals. All these ingredients have a negative effect on the gut environment but also on general health, and when highly processed foods are eaten regularly there is an increased risk of developing chronic diseases associated with poor diet quality such as cardiovascular disease, type-2 diabetes and certain cancers."

The key to good gut health lies not in quick fixes like probiotic drinks or supplements, but increasing overall diversity in your diet. By eating a wide range of plant foods – including some fermented ingredients if you enjoy them – with all their incredible beneficial properties, such as fibre, minerals, vitamins and antioxidants, you'll be giving your gut microbes all the prebiotic foods they like to feed on – as well as topping up all the other ingredients required to ensure the smooth running of a well-oiled human machine.

Tim Spector, Professor of Genetic Epidemiology at King's College, London, and the author of several best-selling books (who is definitely worth following on Instagram @timspector if you're interested in keeping up to date with the latest research into gut health) creates a colourful gardening analogy in his excellent book, *The Diet Myth*. He says: "It's useful to think of your microbial community as your own garden that you are responsible for. We need to make sure the soil (your intestines) that the plants (your microbes) grow in is healthy, containing plenty of nutrients; and to stop weeds or poisonous plants (toxic or disease microbes) taking over we need to cultivate the widest variety of plants and seeds possible ... diversity is the key."[7]

## MINDFUL COOKING AND EATING

Living plantfully is not just about what we eat, it's about how, why and where we eat too. It's all very well deciding to eat more nutrient-rich vegetables, but if your stress levels are through the roof, you tend to eat too quickly or too much, or if you're not enjoying cooking, then you won't enjoy the full benefits. Which is why I don't necessarily think cutting out meat should be your first priority; establishing a happier, healthier way of eating has to start by adopting a new mindset first.

We're all so busy, we don't have time to stop and smell the strawberries, let alone do our food shopping mindfully, but it's this deep disconnection from food that lies at the heart of our health and climate change crises. We don't see first-hand how our food is really produced and the impact this industry has on our environment. Many of us never run our hands through fresh earth to sow seeds or dig up our own potatoes; we never see the vastness of the food waste mountains (other than on a TV documentary), or what it's really like behind the scenes on an intensive livestock farm.

The hectic pace of modern life means we do so much on autopilot. We pick up the same packets at the supermarket every week or just click our "favourites" list doing the online shop, buying things on repeat week in and week out. And while we're cooking, we're trying to supervise the kids' homework or catch up with work emails at the same time. Many meals are eaten "al desko", or in front of the TV, or while scrolling through social media on our phones, so we scoff it down, barely registering what we've just digested. Not to mention all the negative and conflicting messages around food and what we "should" be eating, which sees us going round in a cycle of confusion, self-denial and disappointment as we try out the latest fad diets – and they rarely work. Sound familiar? I know I'm guilty of doing all these things.

The mindless way we shop, cook and eat is doing our health and wellbeing absolutely no favours at all. In fact, it's incredibly damaging to us as individuals and to our wider society. This is why the very first step toward developing a healthier relationship with food is to reconnect with where it comes from, to allow ourselves to feel a sense of wonder at what our Earth provides, and put the joy back into cooking and eating. It may sound a bit hippyish, but trust me – it really helps.

Mindfulness and healthy eating naturally go hand in hand. It's when we shop, cook and eat mindlessly that processed foods slip into our diet or calorific snacks get scoffed on the run. Try to keep in mind the mantra:

128

"eat like a Swede". Inspired by the very simple Swedish philosophy of *lagom,* which is all about striking a healthy balance – *lagom* translates as "not too much, not too little". The Swedes very sensibly believe there's no need to feel guilty about indulging in *fika* (coffee and cake) occasionally if they eat well most of the time. By cooking and eating more mindfully and reconnecting with your appetite, rather than eating through boredom, habit or stress, you will naturally improve your relationship with food.

Anna Jones is one of my favourite food writers, and all her plant-based cookbooks are beautiful and inspirational – a celebration of what she describes as "joyful eating with no tags or labels". I first interviewed Anna around the time of the launch of her third cookbook, *The Modern Cook's Year,* and I remember she said something that really resonated – and it still does. "Even a moment of mindfulness – enjoying the smell of a freshly cut lemon or taking the time to notice the pattern inside a sliced tomato – can be a wonderful thing if you don't have a whole day to languish in the kitchen."

My best advice is to reframe cooking and see it not as yet another chore, but an opportunity to switch off, to unwind, and take pleasure in little tasks such as slicing vegetables or rolling out pastry. Of course, cooking will sometimes be hurried, and it still has to be done, even when you're really not in the mood, but if you can adopt some mindful cooking techniques then I guarantee you'll start to find a lot more pleasure in the creative process, especially when you start trying new plant-based recipes.

# 5 STEPS TO MINDFUL COOKING

1. Try to see the process of discovering different techniques and experimenting with new ingredients as part of the learning process around food that started when you were a child – an education that never stops. Bring a sense of that childlike wonder to new discoveries and see this as an exciting opportunity to eat more delicious, interesting and nutritious foods.

2. Use half an hour in the kitchen to practise being "in the moment". Put aside your phone, put on some relaxing background music and try to anchor your mind to focus exclusively on the task at hand. Tune into all your senses and enjoy the aroma, texture, sound and sight of the food you are preparing.

3. Repetitive tasks such as chopping and stirring can be surprisingly calming. Stop replaying the events of a stressful day or running through your mental to-do list for tomorrow, and focus entirely on slicing your carrots neatly.

4. Don't rush as this causes stress. Assemble all your ingredients, prep all your veg and get your pans ready first. Then start to cook and you'll have time to notice and appreciate each stage of the process using all your senses, from the caramelizing of onions to the aromatic toasting of spices.

5. Cook together. Get your children, teenagers, partner, flatmates or friends involved and make it a social activity. Set tasks such as peeling, chopping or stirring, discuss the ingredients, share new techniques, encourage them to flick through your cookbooks and find other recipes to try. Start having conversations about food and make some mealtimes a collaborative event, with food to share and enjoy – not just a chore.

To reinvent your cooking, you also need to create the right environment and make it more of a pleasure than a chore. Taking a good look at your kitchen and the tools you use every day to prepare food can be a great way to rediscover your mojo. Here are the three things I suggest you do to get your kitchen ready for some creative cooking.

## DECLUTTER YOUR CUPBOARDS

Do you hate getting your food processor out because it's stuck at the back of a high cupboard? Are your worktops covered in clutter? A ruthless audit of your storage and work surface space, to give yourself space to be creative and make your most-used appliances and equipment more accessible, can immediately make cooking more enjoyable.

## INVEST IN QUALITY KNIVES

When you eat more plant foods, the amount of chopping increases exponentially and a knife that feels good in your hand and is properly sharpened makes prep a pleasure. Invest in a good-quality knife, treat it well, hand wash it only and sharpen it regularly and it will last for many years. It's better to have one fabulous knife than a matching set of bog-standard ones, so go for a versatile all-purpose chef's knife and maybe add to your set with a smaller paring and a bread knife later.

## APPLIANCE UPGRADE

Could a new piece of equipment make cooking easier or more efficient? Appliances do take up space, but labour-saving devices such as a kettle-style worktop soupmaker, a slow cooker or a breadmaker enable you to cook from scratch while you're getting on with work or family life elsewhere. A high-speed blender and a decent food processor are both indispensable in my kitchen for making plant-based basics like hummus and nut butter. Save money by looking for second-hand appliances, many of which can be picked up cheaply in pristine condition.

# THE PLANT—BASED BURGER REVOLUTION

Now we come to the business of reducing meat-eating. When people try to cut their intake of meat and fish, often the first thing they do is make simple swaps, such as using veggie sausages for hot dogs at a barbecue. It's a good way to start, especially for those who enjoy the taste and texture of meat but have chosen to reduce their intake or give it up for health, ethical or environmental reasons. With a growing interest in the benefits of a plant-based lifestyle, there's a raft of new meat-style products with an incredibly authentic look and taste, including pies, pizzas, fishless fingers, canned "tuna" and kebab "meat".

The problem is that, unless you're a keen cook, you can become too reliant on convenience products when you first go plant-based and many of these products are packed with sugar, salt and additives. From a nutritional perspective, some meat substitutes are better than others – although some may be more beneficial for our health than you might expect. I spoke to Azmina Govindji, dietitian and author of *Vegan Savvy*, an accessible guide to plant-based nutrition, to get some expert insight. "My research into meat substitutes did really surprise me," says Azmina. "I didn't have high hopes for them nutritionally, but actually I found that some foods based on tempeh, seitan and tofu provide a digestible source of good-quality protein, and can be very valuable in a vegan diet. Ideally, I'd recommend you buy the plainest versions of these foods and add your own flavours, but if you're going to buy more processed products, just keep an eye on the labels for additives, salt, sugar and saturated fat content."

Finding suitable swaps for the meat on the plate without always resorting to processed products can be tricky, especially if you're factoring in the nutritional quality too, so it's good to know that some plant-based products can be healthier. "Replacement products can in some ways be better for you than the meat-based versions," says Azmina. "For example, if you compare vegan burgers with meat burgers, the vegan ones I analyzed for my *Vegan Savvy* book were typically higher in fibre, and many were rich in quality plant-based protein such as pea or soya protein. They won't, however, give you the same amount of iron or certain vitamins and may still be potentially high in salt. But fat levels can sometimes be lower in vegan burgers, depending on how they are cooked."

Ideally, anyone committed to going vegan needs to start developing a repertoire of new recipes. "You have to find things that are delicious and realistic substitutions for your favourite foods," says Azmina. "You're unlikely to maintain this new way of eating in the long term if you simply swap a chicken breast for a slab of plain tofu. Look for dishes that are tasty, quick and easy to prepare, and this is where some flavourful convenience foods can be really useful, like smoked tofu or frozen edamame beans."

However, while some meat substitutes can be helpful, especially in a transition phase, I'm not a huge fan of relying on the "fake meat" type of products too much in the longer term. News stories about "meat" being grown in labs as a "food of the future" and "bleeding burgers" on vegan menus make me feel rather sad that people would prefer to consume these highly processed products when there are so many delicious natural plant-based protein foods available. They're good for an occasional treat, of course – we all have a craving for a burger and fries sometimes – but I can't help thinking that we are swapping one problem for another by switching from meat and fish – which are at least "natural" and nutritious foods – to ultra-processed products with a long list of nutritionally empty ingredients that have to be added to try and recreate the taste and texture of meat or fish.

The move toward plant-based diets has created an opportunity for food manufacturers – after ruining basic products such as bread for us – to now ruin pulses such as soya beans and peas, which are highly nutritious in their natural state, by splitting them up into their constituent parts, reformulating them and creating ultra-processed products to replace that meat gap on the plate. While it is better for the environment to eat a soya burger than it is to eat factory-farmed beef, and it's better to grow protein crops for human consumption than for animal feed, the huge monoculture of crops such as peas or soya that are used to create these fake meat products is simply not sustainable either. Vegan burgers are not the answer and in the next chapter we explore some of the amazing range of plant-based protein foods that you can use to enhance your diet.

Having said all that, it's easy to see the appeal of fake meat foods. For some people, giving up or even just reducing meat is a huge struggle and having some authentic-looking alternatives fills a gap, psychologically at the very least. It's unrealistic to expect the whole world to go completely vegan – and probably unnecessary from a climate change perspective anyway – but scientific developments could be part of the solution to food insecurity and climate change – for example making meat substitutes with lab-grown fungi or lab-grown meat, or even the emerging trend for 3D-printing meat based on real animal cells or plant proteins. The race is on around the world to culture meats such as beef, pork and chicken from cells harvested from animals (with no slaughter necessary) and create cruelty-free, drug-free, commercially viable and sustainable sources of meat for the future. It's thought that these cultured products may be more widely available to the public within as little as 3–5 years. Singapore opened the door by becoming the first country to approve the sale of cultured meat "chicken bites" produced by US company Eat Just in late 2020. The biggest hurdle companies working in this market face is getting regulatory approval and scaling up production in a way that makes it affordable for the mass market, but two separate studies have shown that with the right level of investment, cultivated meat could be on a par pricewise with conventional meat by 2030.[8] Ick factor aside, cultured meat could certainly save on agricultural land and water use and reduce animal welfare issues.

It's fascinating stuff, but surely what we need is a culture change – not cultured meat? Simply continuing to eat lab-grown or highly processed plant-based versions of burgers, chicken nuggets and pulled pork isn't a route to celebrating vegetables or making plants the star of the plate, and it fails to provide a solution to escalating health issues caused by not eating enough vegetables and over consumption of nutritionally depleted ultra-processed foods. In fact, it only reinforces the idea that there's a meat-shaped hole on the plate that needs to be filled with intensively grown plants fashioned into a meat-like shape and flavoured with dozens of unhealthy additives to recreate the meaty taste instead. Sounds a little bit crazy when you put it like that, doesn't it?

# GLOBAL INSPIRATION

When you start looking for recipe ideas to increase your veg intake, try taking a world tour. Eating out is a wonderful opportunity to try something new without having to cook it yourself, and you can take flavours and ingredients you like back to your own kitchen.

Next time you're picking a restaurant, don't go to your usual pizza place – be more adventurous and try a Persian, Japanese, Indian or Nepalese restaurant instead.

There are many cultures where vegetarian food is celebrated and not seen as a "special diet", and where the cuisine is made more interesting through unique uses of herbs and spices.

Southern Indian food is great for being abundant in both its use of pulses for protein and spices for flavour, and while the Italians may love their meat, they also appreciate the simplicity of fresh, seasonal vegetables and staples such as beans and grains.

Beans are also beloved in Mexico and many Mexican favourites can easily be converted to plant-based versions.

Middle Eastern and Persian cooking is so vibrant with a strong tradition of vegetarian food; or look at Chinese cookbooks for dishes that are naturally dairy-free and packed with veggies.

More unusual cuisines to explore could include rich, flavourful Ethiopian cooking or Japanese dishes, but almost every food culture has signature dishes that are veggie-friendly or adaptable.

# 7 SAVVY SWAPS

## 1 SWAP FRUIT JUICE FOR SMOOTHIES

Juices are fine in moderation but switching to a morning smoothie will ensure you get more fibre and other nutrients. It's best to make them with both fruit and vegetables to reduce the sugar content. Remember that a small 150ml (5fl oz) glass of juice or a smoothie (even a vegetable one) only counts as one of your five a day, no matter how many you drink.

## 2 SWAP SANDWICHES FOR SOUP

Sandwiches are perfectly healthy when made with the right ingredients, but switching to soup for lunch can really help you hit your 10-a-day. It's a great way to include veg you (or the kids) are less keen on, and adding in beans or lentils can make your soup thick and hearty – as well as packing a protein punch. If you're not keen on all the beany textures, you can blend it smooth.

## 3 SWAP FRIES FOR VEGETABLE CHIPS

Cut them into chips and you'll be amazed what veg kids might be willing to eat. Root vegetables such as carrots, celeriac (celery root), parsnips and sweet potatoes tossed in a little olive oil and oven baked are delicious. Add extra flavours such as fresh rosemary or sweet smoked paprika for a tasty twist.

## 4 SWAP BUTTER FOR MASHED VEG

For something more nutritious to spread on toast, try mashed avocado or roasted sweet potato, nut butter (ideally homemade or a brand with no added salt, sugar or palm oil), baba ganoush made with aubergine (eggplant) or a bean spread such as hummus. Adding veg such as roasted beetroot (beets) or roasted red (bell) pepper to hummus makes it even more nourishing.

## 5 SWAP WHOLE VEG FOR GRATED

A great way to sneak extra veg varieties into dishes is to use your grater or food processor. You can used grated veg in meat or veggie burgers, quick fritters and salads. A homemade raw slaw with a simple plant-based yoghurt dressing could easily rack up several different vegetables such as carrots, red and white cabbage, celeriac (celery root), fennel, beetroot (beets), radish and red onion.

## 6 SWAP READYMADE SAUCES FOR HOMEMADE

Cooking curry or pasta sauces from scratch using ingredients such as spices, coconut milk or passata enables you to incorporate so many more goodies, and leave out all the nasties. Blending sauces means you can hide all sorts in a pasta bake, risotto or creamy korma and no one will be the wiser, especially if you make them extra delicious with plenty of herbs or spices.

## 7 SWAP DESSERT FOR FRUIT

Naturally sweet and nutritious, fruit is the perfect finale. Skip processed desserts and sugary yoghurts and serve skewers or platters of fresh fruit – top with seeds, toasted coconut or a drizzle of sweet tahini sauce. Dip orange segments or fresh strawberries into melted dark chocolate and leave to harden, or make "nice" cream using bananas and nut butter (*see* recipe on page 143). For a warm dessert, roast stone fruits such as plums, nectarines or apricots and serve topped with toasted porridge oats, nuts and a spoonful of thick plant-based yoghurt.

Yoghurt bark is also lovely – mix any thick plant-based yoghurt with a light drizzle of maple syrup and ½ teaspoon vanilla extract, then spread over a baking sheet lined with baking paper. Scatter fresh fruit such as berries, chopped mango or peaches across the top, along with some chopped toasted nuts, dark chocolate chips, seeds or toasted coconut chips. Freeze for 2–3 hours, then chop into shards and serve.

# 5 WAYS TO VAMP UP YOUR VEG

Here are five dips, dressings and toppings that will make your vegetables sing.

## DUKKAH

*This is a delicious, aromatic, spiced Middle Eastern nut and seed mix that can be used as a topping for soups, salads, roasted vegetables, hummus – pretty much anything you like. Toasting nuts and seeds really brings out their natural nutty flavours. There are many recipes for dukkah so you can experiment with your favourite nuts, seeds and spices, but here's my usual mix.*

**Makes about 300g (10½ oz) | Cooking time: 15 minutes**

### INGREDIENTS

**150g (5oz) mixed nuts (such as almonds, walnuts and hazelnuts)**

**2 tablespoons sesame seeds**

**2 tablespoons fennel seeds**

**2 tablespoons coriander seeds**

**100g (3½oz) other seeds** (such as pumpkin and sunflower)

**1–2 teaspoons ground cumin**

**a generous sprinkle of salt**

### METHOD

Chop the nuts and dry fry until the nuts are just starting to brown. Add the sesame, fennel and coriander seeds to the pan and brown for a few more minutes. Pour out onto a plate to cool.

Add the other seeds to the empty pan and dry fry until popping and lightly toasted.

Pour the cooled nuts and seeds into the food processor and blitz to a rough mixture (not a powder), then transfer to a bowl and stir through the toasted seeds, ground cumin and salt.

Check the seasoning and store in an airtight container for 2 weeks.

# ROASTED VEG CRUMBLE

*I'm very fond of a savoury crumble, and it's amazing how the simplest crispy topping can transform anything from a tray of roasted veg to a salad or soup into something much more special.*

**Serves 4 as a main course | Cooking time: 30–45 minutes**

## INGREDIENTS

**mixed veg for roasting ([bell] peppers, courgettes [zucchini], sweet potato, red onion and chestnut [cremini] mushrooms),** chopped into bite-sized pieces, enough to fill a roasting tin

**drizzle of olive oil**

**fresh thyme leaves**

**garlic cloves, crushed**

**salt and freshly ground black pepper**

**For the crumble topping:**

**breadcrumbs**

**salt and freshly ground black pepper**

**drizzle of olive oil**

**lemon zest**

**fresh thyme leaves** (you can vary the fresh or dried herbs depending on the dish you are making)

## METHOD

Prepare a tray of veg to roast, then drizzle with olive oil, fresh thyme leaves, crushed garlic and seasoning. Put the veg into the oven to roast at a high temperature.

Meanwhile, prepare your crumble topping. Mix the breadcrumbs with seasoning, a drizzle of olive oil, some lemon zest and fresh thyme leaves.

When the vegetables are around 20 minutes away from being cooked, add the breadcrumb topping and bake until golden and crisp.

### TIP

Adding oats to the crumble mix makes a more rustic topping that's particularly good with a creamy gratin such as leek and potato, or try adding mixed seeds for a crunch. To use as a soup or salad topping (or any dish where the topping isn't baked on but sprinkled on before serving), fry the breadcrumbs in a little oil first, then add your flavourings.

# FRUITY SALSA

*A fresh homemade salsa tastes so much more vibrant than the conventional sloppy tomato variety you get ready-made in jars. I love this sweet–spicy combination.*

**Serves 4 as a side dish | Cooking time: 45 minutes**

## INGREDIENTS

**2 spring onions (scallions)**, sliced

**1 mango**, peeled, pitted and finely chopped

**1 x 400g (14oz) can of sweetcorn**, drained, or the kernels cut from 2–3 ears of fresh corn

**a handful of cherry tomatoes**, finely chopped

**a handful of chopped coriander (cilantro)**

**grated zest of 2 limes**

**½ red chilli**, finely chopped (adjust to your taste for heat)

**salt and freshly ground black pepper**

## METHOD

Combine all the ingredients in a bowl and leave to marinade in the fridge for at least 30 minutes before serving.

This goes well with spicy dishes, salads, bean chilli, fajitas and tacos.

### TIP

Add a can of drained, rinsed black beans to make it more substantial.

# PERI-PERI TAHINI DRESSING

*This simple dressing is great for drizzling over vegetables, falafel and salads.*

**Serves 2 | Cooking time: 5 minutes**

## INGREDIENTS

**2 tablespoons tahini**

**1 garlic clove, crushed**

**juice of ½ lemon**

**½ teaspoon peri-peri seasoning**

**4–5 tablespoons cold water**

## METHOD

Add the tahini, garlic, lemon juice and peri-peri seasoning to a bowl and whisk with the cold water until smooth.

### TIP

For different flavours, switch the peri-peri seasoning for other spice mixes such as Cajun or Baharat.

# ROMESCO SAUCE

*This intense Spanish sauce is so versatile – use it as a dip with flatbreads or vegetable skewers, as a pasta sauce or a jacket potato topping or serve with roast potatoes or Mediterranean vegetables.*

**Serves 2 | Cooking time: 10 minutes**

## INGREDIENTS

**100g (3½oz) blanched almonds**

**2 roasted (bell) peppers**
(roast them yourself or use 2 drained jarred peppers)

**1 garlic clove**, chopped

**1 tablespoon sherry vinegar**
(you could also use red wine or apple vinegar, but using any vinegar is optional)

**1 teaspoon paprika**

**3–4 tablespoons extra virgin olive oil**

## METHOD

Tip the almonds into a dry frying pan (skillet) over a medium-low heat, shaking regularly until they are golden and smell nice and toasty.

Put the roasted peppers into a food processor with the garlic, vinegar (if using) and paprika. Blitz to a textured paste, then gradually add the olive oil to get the consistency you want – use less oil for a thicker sauce for a veg topping or dip, or add more for a thinner sauce for pasta.

# 2 PLANT-PACKED SWEET TREATS

Even desserts and snacks can be rich in healthy plant ingredients, and homemade treats using naturally sweet ingredients such as fresh or dried fruit, nut butters and dark chocolate are good choices as part of a healthy, balanced diet.

## NUTTY BANANA MAPLE NICE CREAM

*For a healthy fruit-based dessert, try this delicious fruit-based dairy-free "nice" cream with minimal sweetener, and nuts for extra goodness. I've also made this without maple syrup and it's still good, providing your bananas are super ripe and sweet.*

**Serves 3–4 | Prep time: 5 minutes (+ freezing time)**

### INGREDIENTS

**5 ripe bananas**

**3 tablespoons unsweetened plant milk**

**1 heaped tablespoon almond or peanut butter**

**1 tablespoon maple syrup** and extra to serve

**chopped walnuts or dark chocolate chips**, to serve

### METHOD

Peel and slice the bananas, then place them on a layer of baking paper on a tray. Pop the tray in the freezer overnight.

Tip the frozen bananas into a high-speed blender with the plant milk, nut butter and maple syrup. Pulse until the mixture is smooth and creamy.

You can eat this immediately – it's very soft like gelato at this point – or freeze it in a lidded container overnight for a more scoopable consistency. To serve, drizzle with maple syrup and scatter with chopped walnuts or chocolate chips.

# CHOCOLATE AND PEANUT BONBONS

*These fabulous little balls of chocolatey and peanutty goodness are so incredibly easy to make. If you have never made an energy ball before, this is a great recipe to start with as everyone loves them. Packed with nutritious ingredients, they are a much better alternative to processed snacks or chocolate and are great for an after-school or post-exercise energy boost.*

**Makes 20 balls | Prep time: 20 minutes**

## INGREDIENTS

**200g (7oz) pitted dates**

**80g (3oz) oats**

**20g (¾oz) mixed seeds**
(I use a mix of pumpkin, sunflower, sesame and brown linseed)

**1 heaped tablespoon Fair Trade cacao powder or unsweetened cocoa powder**

**2 tablespoons unsweetened peanut butter, smooth or crunchy** (or use almond butter, if you prefer)

**40g (1½oz) desiccated (shredded unsweetened) coconut (optional)**

## METHOD

Put the dates in a bowl and soak in hot water for 5–10 minutes until softened.

Place the oats and seeds in a food processor or blender and whizz until finely ground. My food processor is a bit ancient so they keep a bit of texture, which I like, but you can go finer if you prefer.

Drain the dates and thoroughly press out any excess water. Add the dates, cacao powder and peanut butter to the oat and seed mixture and whizz until the mixture forms a thick paste. If it's a bit dry, add a drop of water, just enough to bring the mixture together without it being too wet.

Roll small amounts of the mixture in your hand to form 20 balls.

Scatter the desiccated coconut onto a plate, if using, and roll each ball around the plate until thoroughly coated.

Keep in an airtight container in the fridge for up to a week. They also freeze well – just leave in the fridge overnight or at room temperature for an hour or two before you want to eat them.

# KEEP AN EYE ON YOUR OMEGAS

We all need sources of healthy fats in our diet; it's essential for many processes in the body, from forming cell walls to brain development, plus it ensures we can absorb essential fat-soluble nutrients such as vitamins A, D and E.

Omega 6 fatty acids are needed for making many enzymes the body uses to build and regulate our immune and inflammatory systems, and omega 3s are now known to be crucial for reducing inflammation – and deficiencies have been linked to conditions such as arthritis, heart disease and dementia. Oily fish are the best natural sources of omega 3 fatty acids, along with fortified eggs; those found in plant foods are not as readily available to the body and are not considered to be as heart-healthy as those from fish. If your diet is fully plant-based, ensure your diet includes plenty of healthy fats such as extra virgin rapeseed, extra virgin olive, avocado and hemp oils, plus nuts and seeds such as walnuts, flaxseeds, hemp seeds, chia seeds, pumpkin seeds and nut butters, along with foods such as seaweed, avocado and edamame beans.

Many of us consume far too much omega 6 and not enough omega 3. To help rectify this, processed foods and oils, which typically contain higher levels of omega 6, or saturated fats such as coconut, palm, sesame, sunflower, soyabean and corn oil should be used sparingly.

You could add a vegan algae-based supplement to your diet as a back-up – nori, chlorella and spirulina (the latter is also rich in essential amino acids) can be farmed sustainably.

145

## SIGNPOSTS

For more on:

- ❀ The Planetary Health Diet, *see* chapter 2
- ❀ Inflammation, *see* chapters 1 and 2
- ❀ Gut health, *see* chapter 3 and 7
- ❀ Plant-based protein, *see* chapter 8
- ❀ Herbs, *see* chapter 4
- ❀ Growing your own vegetables, *see* chapter 3

# 8

# GIVE PEAS (BEANS AND GRAINS) A CHANCE

"The Gods created certain kinds of beings to replenish our bodies; they are the trees and the plants and the seeds."

Plato

**THE GOAL:
TO POWER UP WITH PLANT PROTEIN**

**I**'M GOING TO COME RIGHT OUT AND ADMIT THAT BEANS
and lentils have something of an image problem. I don't think I'll ever
forget my first experience of lentil loaf at our local "health food café" in
the 1980s, which was Sahara-dry and without even a glimmer of flavour.
But meat-free food has come a very long way since then, so don't dismiss
pulses because of previous bad experiences; they are hero ingredients in
a plant-based diet and are not only deliciously healthy for us – they also
naturally improve the fertility of the soil by enriching it with nitrogen as they
grow too.

There's almost an embarrassment of riches to write about when it comes
to the nutritional and health benefits of pulses. But it's not enough to know
pulses are good for us – it's delicious flavours and exciting recipes that
inspire us to try and keep eating new foods. It took a while for this to click
for me, but you can use pulses in absolutely everything, including sweet
and savoury dishes, and you don't even need to have a specific recipe for
beans or lentils, especially if you are using pre-cooked varieties from a tin or
pouch. Every time I make a soup, a pasta dish, a tray of roasted vegetables
or a curry, I chuck a can of beans or lentils in too, letting them soak up all
the lovely flavours and bring their distinctive texture to the mix. Including
a wide variety of beans, pulses and grains in meals throughout the week will
also help you hit your 30 different plant foods target.

Although rich in protein, beans are not a straightforward switch with meat
on the plate. Swapping a steak for a pile of kidney beans isn't going to
be very appetizing even for the most ardent bean lover, so you do have
to get a little creative. But their star feature in a dish when used whole is
texture, and this is something often missing from plant-based dishes that
only contain vegetables. They are brilliant for adding a more substantial
mouthfeel to veggie dishes and this texture, which most types of beans
and lentils hold onto well even after cooking, makes them ideally suited
to making recipes such as veggie burgers. They are also great for making
creamy soups, sauces and dips, and are an economical way to bulk out both
meat and veggie dishes to make them stretch further.

Most plain beans, lentils and bean-based products such as tofu have only a
mild beany, slightly earthy flavour, so they need to be enhanced with other

ingredients to achieve their full potential. This is where herbs, spices, full-flavoured sauces and long, slow cooking methods such as stews or oven bakes will really bring out the best in pulses.

## THE PROTEIN MYTH

We've all become a bit obsessed with protein lately. Manufacturers have latched onto the trend, promoting everything from sliced bread to granola bars as "high-protein" foods to make them more appealing to health-conscious consumers – even though they probably have no more protein in them than they did before they were repackaged.

It's partly down to a number of studies suggesting that eating more protein may help us achieve a healthier weight or perform better at sport. It's true that a high-protein diet can help build lean muscle, in combination with exercise, and lean muscle helps to burn more calories throughout the day. Protein also tends to make us feel fuller for longer, so we're less likely to scoff unhealthy snacks, which is part of the reason it's hailed as a hero nutrient for dieters.

## NUTRITIONAL NOTE

High in protein, fibre and B vitamins while low in fat and calories, pulses contribute to one portion of your five a day (80g/3oz or 3 heaped tablespoons). Combining pulses with grains and vitamin C-rich foods enhances their protein content and enables the body to better absorb their iron and other nutrients.

Packed with antioxidants that can reduce inflammation and help prevent chronic diseases such as cancer, pulses also promote bone health, while the phytoestrogens particularly prevalent in soya beans, can also reduce cognitive decline and help with menopause symptoms.

But this isn't the purpose of protein, more a beneficial side effect. One of the main macronutrients in our diet, alongside carbohydrate and fat, protein is needed mainly for building and repairing body cells, and making enzymes, hormones and antibodies. As new studies continually reveal, the secret to achieving a healthy weight is much more complex – not to mention genetically, environmentally and individually determined – than simply getting that elusive perfect balance of macros in your diet.

Protein's star has risen thanks to the popularity of low-carb diets too, with people often lumping all carbohydrates together in the "bad" camp, when in fact complex carbohydrates such as wholegrains, pulses and vegetables are an equally important part of a balanced diet. Protein and carbohydrates contain the same 4 kcals per gram – it's just that our carb portion sizes tend to be more generous, so they often seem heavier on the calories. Carbs are your body's main source of fuel, and because protein plays such an important role in maintaining healthy muscles and bones, you need to have a good supply of complex carbs to meet your body's energy needs or it will start wasting your protein intake by using it for energy. This is especially important if you are very sporty and active.

The only carbs we need to cut down on are the highly processed varieties that have had all the fibre, vitamins and minerals stripped away, such as white bread, sugary cereals, processed cakes and biscuits and white pasta, which trigger rapid spikes in blood sugar and insulin after eating, quickly followed by an energy crash and a return of hunger. These refined foods have been associated with an increased tendency for overeating and are linked with obesity, heart disease and diabetes.

Pulses and wholegrains, on the other hand, are nutritious packages that contain both carbohydrates and protein and are linked with lower rates of those same harmful lifestyle diseases. In fact, some foods that are generally considered to be in the carb camp may be higher in protein than you might expect – for example, oats and some types of vegetables. It's a useful reminder that we get our protein intake from a wide range of sources and not always the obvious ones, particularly in a plant-based diet.

When people announce they're going veggie or vegan, one of the first questions they're often asked is "Will you get enough protein?" But have you ever thought about where the animals we eat get their protein from? It comes from the soil, via the plants they eat. It's perfectly possible for us to cut out the middleman and just eat protein-rich plants directly ourselves. Pulses, nuts, seeds and grains are surprisingly rich protein sources, and plant foods such as tofu, tempeh (both made from soya beans), peas, nuts, hemp seeds and lentils provide high-quality complete protein just like meat.

A high-quality protein contains adequate amounts of all nine essential amino acids, while a lesser-quality protein does not have the full range of amino acids, which is another good reason to eat a wide variety of grains, pulses, vegetables, seeds and nuts.

Anita Bean, registered nutritionist and author of several books on vegetarian and vegan nutrition, agrees variety is key. "Focusing on plant-based sources of protein has ethical advantages, of course, but also may improve our health and wellbeing, as many plant sources of protein are naturally lower in saturated fat and calories than meat products, and many also have other benefits such as being higher in fibre. However, while plant foods such as soya, quinoa and hemp seeds are complete proteins, most plant-based foods don't contain all the essential amino acids we need, which is why it's particularly important if you're veggie or vegan to enjoy a balanced diet with a wide variety of protein-rich foods."

Some people do gain weight when they first go plant-based, but that's usually because they fill up on too many processed foods or carbohydrates instead, turning to things like bread, pasta or baked potatoes. This is where plant protein foods such as beans, lentils, tofu, nuts and seeds are so important for filling that gap, satisfying hunger while supplying plenty of other important nutrients and micronutrients. A well-planned, balanced plant-based diet usually leads to people losing a few pounds and achieving a healthier weight.

So how much protein do we actually need? The average person requires a minimum of 0.8g protein per kilogram of body weight a day, although this can increase to 2g if you're a regular exerciser or are trying to lose fat and prevent muscle loss. Because the proteins from plants appear to be less digestible than meat protein, if you're eating predominantly plant-based, it's a good idea to aim for a slightly higher intake, especially if you are very physically active or over 60. Around 20g of protein at every meal plus a protein-rich snack every day is a good target to aim for. Most of us haven't a clue what 20g protein looks like on the plate, but it's really not difficult to rack it up if you ensure you use beans, pulses, nuts, seeds and wholegrains in every meal. For example:

- A snack of 80g (3oz) chickpea (garbanzo bean) hummus with 2 oatcakes is 10g protein.

- Half a can of baked beans on two large slices of wholegrain bread is 20g.

- A large bowl of porridge oats (50g/2oz) made with 300ml (10fl oz) soya milk and topped with 2 tablespoons pumpkin seeds is 20g.

So, while you'll want to think about upping your intake of protein-rich plant foods, there's no need to fret too much about it – very few people in the developed world have a deficiency of protein, and many of us eat as much as 50% more protein than we actually need.

# THE BEST FOODS TO TOP UP YOUR PLANT-BASED PROTEIN

While exotic ingredients such as blue-green algae, teff and hemp powder are certainly great sources of this important macronutrient, you don't have to buy supplements or vegan protein powders to get your RDA of protein, as there's plenty to be found in these everyday food sources.

## SOYA YOGHURT

Unsweetened soya yoghurt is protein-rich and low in fat.

## BEANS, PEAS AND LENTILS

All beans, peas and lentils are a low-fat and budget-friendly way to boost your protein intake, along with fibre and other benefits too. Whether you choose fresh edamame, canned black beans, dried red lentils or frozen green peas, most contain 5–9g protein per 100g (3½oz) cooked, and even baked beans count – ideally choose no- or low-sugar and salt varieties. Combine pulses with some nuts to get a complete protein fix.

## NUTS AND SEEDS

Whether you add them to your granola, toss a handful into your stir-fry, have nut butter on toast for lunch (ideally choose 100% nut butters with no added oil, salt or sugar) or make chia pudding for dessert, nuts and seeds are an easy way to perk up your protein levels. You don't need to consume loads to get the benefits – hemp seeds contain 5g per heaped tablespoon, chia seeds offer 2g per tablespoon and there's 4g in 6 Brazil nuts.

## QUINOA, BUCKWHEAT AND AMARANTH

A complete protein, quinoa seeds contain all eight essential amino acids. Use it as you would couscous or rice or mix with other grains. If you aren't keen on the taste or texture, try using quinoa flakes in muesli or porridge instead. Amaranth and buckwheat are pseudo grains that can be used in much the same way as quinoa and are both rich in fibre and protein – they also come in flakes and flour form.

## TOFU AND TEMPEH

Soya is one of the best plant sources of protein and contains all the amino acids we need from food. Tofu is essentially pressed soya bean curd and is rich in iron, calcium and essential minerals. Use firm tofu cubed in dishes such as stir-fries or curries or blend silken tofu into soups, sauces and desserts. Tempeh is another soya bean product – but in this case it is fermented and pressed – producing a denser, chewier texture that makes it "meatier" in texture, making it ideal as a vegan burger, for example. As a fermented food, tempeh is rich in probiotics, which are good for gut health, and it's also high in protein and nutrients such as magnesium, phosphorus and manganese. However, it's quite calorie-dense, so watch your portion size.

## VEGETABLES

Although veggies are often overlooked as a protein source, you may be surprised to discover that they still pack a punch – with asparagus offering almost 2g protein in every 6 spears and broccoli around 3g per 100g (3½oz), and even sweetcorn provides over 2g in 3 heaped tablespoons. With many veggies containing some protein, if you ensure you eat a range of produce every day, including plenty of greens and brassicas such as broccoli and cauli, you'll naturally be getting plenty of plant protein.

## MYCOPROTEIN

Made from a slightly unappetizing-sounding "mycoprotein", which originates from an edible, natural fungus, the surprisingly tasty end result – often marketed as Quorn – has long been one of the most popular meat substitute brands on the market, offering everything from mince to sausages, bacon and chicken-style pieces. It is high in protein – 14g per 100g (3½oz) – and is also high in fibre and low in saturated fat, so if your family enjoys classic dishes with meat-style alternatives, then this is not a bad choice from a nutritional perspective. If you want to be strictly plant-based, not all Quorn products are vegan, so do check labels.

## SEITAN

Made from wheat gluten and water, seitan is another meat alternative with an authentically "meaty" texture and is a good option for those who can't eat soya. Seitan also contains iron and selenium, but store-bought varieties can be highly processed with additives, salt and preservatives – so do check labels or make your own at home.

## PLUS ... A NOTE ON JACKFRUIT AND BANANA BLOSSOM

Jackfruit (a large tropical fruit with a shredded flesh inside) and banana blossom (a south-east Asian fleshy, purple-skinned flower that grows at the end of the banana fruit) have become quite popular in vegan recipes lately. Unripe jackfruit does a great job of mimicking pulled pork and other meaty dishes when cooked with the right spices, while banana blossom has a chunky, flaky texture reminiscent of fish and tastes pretty good when battered and served with chips and vegan tartare sauce. However, neither are really a good protein substitute, so it's best to add ingredients such as beans, quinoa or lentils to boost the protein content.

## COOKING WITH PULSES AND GRAINS

When you first start using beans and lentils, it's often easier to buy pre-cooked varieties in cans, ideally organic. If you can find them, beans such as chickpeas (garbanzos) and butterbeans (lima) in jars (usually found in delis and health-food stores) are often better quality. Pre-cooked pouches of interesting grains, Puy lentils and grain-and-bean mixes are a no-faff option. They tend to be more expensive and may have added extras such as oil or salt, but they are a good way to try something new or for a quick fix when time is tight.

If you start using beans and pulses regularly, it's more economical to buy them dried and batch-cook them yourself. You can keep some to use fresh and freeze the rest. Soaking dried grains and pulses with longer cooking times can reduce the time required (saving on energy too) – you can either leave them to soak in cold water overnight before cooking, or bring the pot to the boil, lid on, then remove from the heat and leave for an hour to soak. Then add seasoning and boil as normal. Some people believe soaking reduces the phytate content of pulses that can hinder mineral absorption to some extent, and also makes beans more digestible and less likely to cause bloating and wind, although gut health experts say that introducing pulses gradually and then eating them regularly to allow the good gut bacteria that can digest them properly to flourish is the key to avoiding any unpleasant digestive effects. Whether you pre-soak or not comes down to individual preference.

Quinoa does not need to be soaked but should be thoroughly rinsed before cooking to remove the slightly soapy flavour.

Toasting and popping grains in a dry pan or roasting them in the oven for 5 minutes until they are golden before cooking as normal is a great way to bring out the naturally nutty flavours.

# 7 WAYS TO PACK IN PULSES

1.  **Hummus-style bean dips** Not just good for chips and dips, hummus and other bean purées can be used instead of butter or mayo in sandwiches, to top baked potatoes or as a topping for dishes such as veggie chilli or nachos.

2.  **Soup** This is a really easy way to enjoy some "hidden" pulses. I like to add red lentils (which don't hold their shape in cooking like brown, green and Puy do) to red soups (for example, tomato, butternut squash, sweet potato) and add a kick of spices such as curry paste or smoky paprika. For pale or green soups, such as celeriac (celery root), parsnip, leek or peas, I find blending in butterbeans (lima beans) along with woody herbs such as thyme makes a creamy, aromatic soup.

3.  **Dhal** Cheap to make and super healthy, dhal is such a lovely introduction to lentils, and this soothing dish can be enjoyed instead of soup for lunch, or served with a wholegrain for a main meal. Stir in lots of fresh herbs and baby spinach leaves at the end of cooking for extra flavour and goodness.

4.  **Adding texture** Beans and firmer green and brown lentils are brilliant for adding texture and substance to homemade veggie burgers to serve in a bun with all the trimmings, or no-meat balls to go with pasta and a rich tomato sauce. They're also brilliant to replace or bulk out the meat in pasta sauces, lasagne, moussaka and curries.

5.  **Baking** Beans really work in baking and are especially good for making gluten-free treats that use less added oil or butter. Ideal for anyone not a big fan of their taste and texture, beans are barely detectable in most baked goods. There are lots of recipes out there for white beans in cakes, while chocolate cakes and brownies work well with black beans.

6.  **Smoothies** Another idea for those not so keen on their flavour or texture, white beans can be added to smoothies to add a thick, creamy texture and a protein punch. This is a great way to thicken smoothies if you don't always want to use banana.

7. **Creamy Sauces** You can blend cooked white beans such as cannellini, butterbeans (lima beans), split peas or split fava beans with stock, seasoning, nutritional yeast and your choice of herbs to create creamy sauces for pasta or for layering in dishes such as veggie lasagne or lentil moussaka.

# GOOD FOR YOU, GOOD FOR THE PLANET

Changing up our grains occasionally not only brings fresh new flavours and textures into our diet, but if more of us make the switch regularly it also creates a demand for more sustainable, more nutritious, locally grown grain and pulse crops, which farmers and retailers will respond to.

We already have many under-appreciated ancient grains to turn to, and some farmers are seeing the potential for growing traditional varieties. Josiah Meldrum, co-founder of pioneering pulse brand Hodmedod, which produces unusual and some globally scarce pulse and grains, says: "When we founded Hodmedod, we looked at how to make better economic and agro-ecological returns for farms, with lower chemical inputs and more space for considering biodiversity. Along with pulses, that included crops such as chia and camelina (a small seed from the brassica family) and quinoa, along with higher value, old fashioned and under-utilized cereals that have a more interesting and valuable nutritional profile than modern wheat."

Among more unusual beans such as carlin peas (a great alternative to chickpeas/garbanzos) or split fava beans (traditionally used to make Ta'amia, a type of Egyptian falafel), Hodmedod also produces landrace wheats and ancient grains such as emmer (known as farro when eaten as a wholegrain) and einkorn.

"We're big fans of naked barley, which is a very easily digestible, high beta-glucan barley that doesn't require polishing," says Josiah. "We also produce naked oats, which don't need to be hulled – a process that requires a high level of mechanization that can't be done on a small scale. Naked oats are higher in oil and good fat content and make a delicious and nutritious alternative to brown long grain rice."

The beauty of switching grains is that most are easily interchangeable – almost any grain will work in a pilaf or a grain salad, and if served with stews or curries most will do a great job of mopping up all those lovely sauces. Just grab a bag of something different and try a few recipes with it. Mixing beans in with your grains increases the quality of protein in a dish too.

- At breakfast, swap conventional oats in porridge, muesli or granola for quinoa, amaranth or millet flakes. Make bircher muesli pots with buckwheat, kamut or farro instead of oats, and top with fresh berries.

- Rather than always reaching for wheat flour, make pancakes with buckwheat or oat flour; use emmer or spelt flour to make bread or try buckwheat or spelt flour for cakes.

- For risotto, in place of rice, use spelt, teff, buckwheat, kamut or pearl barley, or for pilaf use quinoa, wheat berries, barley, spelt, freekeh or farro. Try any of these grains for serving with curries and chillies.

- Make hearty grain salads with quinoa, amaranth, farro, freekeh or bulgur wheat. Add lots of raw or roasted vegetables, fresh herbs, beans, nuts and seeds with a delicious dressing.

- Switch up your grains in family favourites – veggie burgers, fritters or falafels can be made with added cooked quinoa, buckwheat, bulgur wheat or farro. Instead of pasta bake, try spelt or farro with a rich herby tomato sauce, beans, vegetables and some veggie sausages.

## TOPPING UP YOUR TANK

Iron is needed to make the protein haemoglobin, which transports oxygen in red blood cells to all the cells in the body. An iron deficiency can mean a reduction in haemoglobin and less oxygen to supply your body's needs, which can cause fatigue. If you're new to plant-based eating and start to feel tired all the time, it might be a good idea to take a look at your iron intake.

There are plenty of everyday plant foods that provide iron, including fortified cereals and oats, tempeh, pumpkin seeds, quinoa, wholegrain bread, beans and pulses, tahini and nut butters, and dried fruits, but plant iron (non-haem) is less well-absorbed than animal-derived iron (haem iron), which comes directly from the haemoglobin protein in the animal's cells. Tea and coffee can also hamper absorption, so avoid drinking them with meals.

Vitamin C helps to convert iron into a more usable form, but it must be consumed at the same meal. So, for example, if you are having a bowl of iron-fortified porridge for breakfast, top it with fresh strawberries or at lunch enjoy a spinach salad with slices of orange and a sprinkle of pumpkin seeds. If you aim to serve every meal with a salad of colourful vegetables, a small glass of fruit juice (unsweetened and only once a day because of the naturally high sugar content), or a piece of fruit for dessert, as well as always adding a rainbow of veg to your cooked dishes, your iron levels should be adequate.

# HOW TO MAKE TOFU TASTE AMAZING

Tofu is a fantastic ingredient, but it needs to be prepared properly to taste great. You can buy ready-marinated and smoked tofu for extra flavour or add your own spices, marinades and sauces.

**Buy the Right Type**
For savoury cooking, always look for firm or extra-firm tofu. Silken tofu is softer and usually used for dishes such as desserts and sauces.

**Crisp It Up**
If you are dry stir-frying or roasting and would like a crispy finish, lightly coat the tofu in cornflour (cornstarch) first, then dust in your choice of dry spices (Chinese five spice is good) and stir fry or roast in a little oil for crispy, tasty cubes.

**Press It**
Pressing tofu to remove as much moisture as possible before cooking also helps it absorb more flavour and crisp up better,

although if you are using it in liquid sauces such as curries or braises, there's no need to press it. You can use a tofu press or simply wrap it in a clean tea (dish) towel or kitchen paper and put it between two chopping boards with something heavy on top to give it a good squeeze for 30 minutes.

### Marinate It

Here's my favourite way to cook tofu. Make a marinade of 2 finely chopped garlic cloves, 2 tablespoons tamari, 1 tablespoon nutritional yeast and a grinding of freshly ground black pepper. Add 200g (7oz) plain firm tofu cut into cubes and leave to soak up the flavours for 30 minutes. Don't add oil to marinades as this can hamper flavour absorption. Transfer to a baking dish, drizzle with rapeseed (canola) oil and bake in the oven at a moderate heat for 20 minutes, turning once. Serve dressed with a few drops of sesame oil and toasted sesame seeds. This is lovely served with some stir-fried greens.

## SIGNPOSTS

For more on:

🌱 How pulses improve soil health, *see* chapter 2

🌱 Chickpeas, *see* chapter 9

🌱 Easy ways to eat more plants, *see* chapter 7

# 9

# IS THERE ANYTHING CHICKPEAS CAN'T DO?

"vegetarian and frugal it may be, but the chickpea is one of the most versatile ingredients you could keep in your cupboards."

Yotam Ottolenghi

**THE GOAL:**
**TO FIND EXCITING ALTERNATIVES TO EGGS**

**A**LL PULSES ARE PRETTY AMAZING LITTLE PARCELS OF GOODNESS, but if I had to pick one favourite in my kitchen it would have to be chickpeas, aka garbanzo beans. Hummus is probably the most famous chickpea-based recipe on the planet and the UK alone gets through 12,000 tonnes of this rather beige, unassuming, yet incredibly delicious dip every year. With slightly mysterious "Middle Eastern" origins, everyone from the Turks to the Syrians, Greeks, Israelis and the Lebanese have tried to claim it. The latter sparked the "hummus wars" in 2008, when the Lebanon petitioned (and failed) to get the EU to officially recognize hummus as a Lebanese dish. The origins are as mysterious as the correct spelling (hummus or houmous?) and the definitive recipe – everyone has their own variation, although chickpeas, tahini, lemon juice and extra virgin olive oil are the essentials for any authentic hummus.

What isn't in question is how much we love it. Hummus is delicious, yet also cheap, nutritious and versatile. It's considered equally acceptable to serve it to children with carrot sticks at teatime, or to drizzle a little pomegranate molasses on top, add some flatbreads to make a mezze dish for a smart soirée.

Humans have been cultivating nutritious, fibre- and protein-rich chickpeas for well over 7,000 years – some sources say 10,000 years in Turkey – and they were one of the first cultivated pulse crops. They remain one of the most popular pulses across the globe too, and from India to the Middle East, Europe to Africa they are consumed in vast quantities, putting them in the top twenty crops grown worldwide. But for many people today, hummus is still their only contact with the chickpea – or with pulses generally – and that's a shame, because they're a rather magical and versatile little bean, and one of their most interesting uses in the plant-based kitchen is, rather surprisingly, as an egg replacement.

# NUTRITIONAL NOTE

Chickpeas are low in calories and have a low GI, which means they help stabilize blood sugar levels, while their soluble fibre content helps maintain healthy gut and bowel function. Studies have shown that people who eat chickpeas regularly are less likely to be overweight. One study of Australian women revealed that participants were less likely to eat junk food when they ate around 100g (3½oz) chickpeas a day for 12 weeks,[1] suggesting that including this pulse in your diet may keep you feeling fuller for longer and make it easier to maintain a healthy weight.

Although chickpeas are an excellent source of plant-based protein and contain almost all the essential amino acids we need, try to serve chickpeas with some wholegrains to get the full range.

## GOOD FOR YOU, GOOD FOR THE PLANET

We eat billions of eggs every year. The environmental impact of eggs is higher than plant foods but much lower than meat, especially beef. If you're comparing sources of protein for the most eco-friendly options, 50g (2oz) of protein from 7 large eggs has a carbon footprint almost 12 times less than 50g (2oz) of protein from one small beef steak (190g/6½oz, raised on deforested land).[2]

Most of the carbon impact of eggs comes from the farming process rather than packaging or transport; raising the chickens and growing their feed releases substantial amounts of carbon dioxide and nitrous oxide into the atmosphere globally. Ironically, a study from Cranfield University suggests organic eggs would be 25% worse for climate change than those from battery farms.[3] It's an interesting example of how the solutions to the climate crisis are never straightforward, although after researching the animal welfare issues of the egg industry for this book I'd strongly recommend that if you are going to eat eggs, you should prioritize higher ethical standards and buy organic regardless.

So, should we reduce or give up eggs completely? The EAT-*Lancet's* Planetary Health Diet recommends dramatically reducing individual egg intake to 13g (about ½oz) a week, which works out at a rather awkward one and a half eggs – maybe more sensibly this could equate to one egg one week, two the next. Either way, it's low based on our current rate of egg eating.

Eggs are also hidden away in a huge variety of readymade products, including cakes, noodles, dressings and bread, and egg-eating statistics include the invisible eggs we eat in many kinds of sweet and savoury processed foods. However, such eggs are the biggest ethical concern, because those used in processed foods are rarely high welfare, free range or organic.

If you are heading toward plant-centred eating and are thinking about reducing or eliminating eggs, the humble chickpea is your go-to alternative for making everything from mayonnaise to meringues. For egg replacement, gram (aka besan or chickpea) flour and aquafaba are two very useful ingredients:

## AQUAFABA
This is the liquid from cans or jars of chickpeas, which can be whipped like egg whites to make recipes such as vegan meringues and mousses – pretty impressive for a by-product that usually gets poured down the drain.

## GRAM FLOUR (BESAN)
This is made from dried, ground chickpeas and is ideal for making batters in traditional eggy dishes such as pancakes and quiche fillings.

Not only do they work miracles in the kitchen, but chickpeas also have a carbon footprint substantially lower than eggs. In fact, chickpeas, like all pulses, have one of the lowest carbon footprints of any food group, and as they are "nitrogen fixers" they not only enrich our diet, they also improve soil quality by restoring nitrogen to the earth without the need for chemical fertilizers, which is just one of many reasons why pulses are the plant-based proteins of the future.

# SIZE MATTERS

If you do use eggs, never buy large or extra-large varieties as this causes pain and health problems for hens. The yolks are the same size regardless of the size of the egg and smaller eggs are also more likely to be laid by younger hens in their prime and are generally tastier. The best option is to buy boxes of "mixed weight" eggs, which reflects the natural variety of what hens produce.

In recipes that call for large eggs, switch 2 large eggs for 3 medium, or stick to 2 eggs and add a splash of milk if the recipe needs more moisture. When making meringues, you should weigh the egg whites and double the weight in sugar.

In most recipes you can use one of the egg-replacement methods I've suggested on page 164.

The British Hen Welfare Trust provides more information at www.bhwt.org.uk

## HOW TO REPLACE EGGS IN THE KITCHEN

In cooking, eggs are often used to fulfil a practical purpose in a recipe, such as binding ingredients together or adding a light, airy texture. Experimental cooks have proved eggs are not as irreplaceable as we once thought, and there are plenty of interesting egg alternatives you can try.

There are a variety of commercial egg replacement products on the market, usually containing ingredients such as potato starch, arrowroot and tapioca starch that emulsify, moisten and bind like eggs. However, I prefer to replace eggs with more natural ingredients wherever possible and, depending on the recipe, there are lots of different options. Remember that some of these replacements may require a little trial and error to get the taste and texture right in your favourite recipes, but often the egg-free versions exceed the deliciousness of the original egg-based versions – so have fun experimenting.

# BAKING

To replace eggs and milk or buttermilk in baking, try switching with 60g (2oz) soya or coconut yoghurt per egg, which gives a slightly sour taste and light texture, especially good for muffins, scones and soda bread. For a great rise add ¼ teaspoon bicarbonate of soda (baking soda). Carbonated water can also give a good rise to cakes, so switch one egg for 60ml (2fl oz) sparkling water.

Fresh and dried fruit can also work in puddings such as cakes, brownies, fruit loaf, pancakes and muffins. Try substituting 60g (2oz) mashed banana, apple purée, sweet potato, avocado, butternut squash or soaked puréed dates for one egg, which add different levels of flavour and sweetness. They work well as binders, giving a moist texture to your baking, although adding too much can make your bake dense and heavy and can affect the flavour, so you may need to experiment with the quantities. The same goes for 60g (2oz) puréed silken tofu, which is a protein-rich egg replacement that can also result in a denser bake, so avoid using for anything that should be light and fluffy.

While puréed fruits and veg or tofu can work well in "squidgier" bakes like brownies and muffins, they usually won't be suitable for recipes that should be crisp, such as biscuits or cookies. A commercial egg replacer is often the best option here – or choose a recipe that doesn't use eggs in the first place. You could also try using 60g (2oz) of a creamy smooth nut butter, such as almond, cashew or peanut, in biscuits (it may also work for pancakes and brownies too) to replace one egg.

As a general rule, if you're adapting a recipe it's best not to use these methods in any that call for three eggs or more. All these replacements may involve trial and error, so if you're not an experienced baker, start with something simple or look for vegan recipes. There are some great vegan cake recipes out there that use tactics such as adding extra bicarbonate of soda (baking soda) and some lemon juice mixed with plant milk to make a deliciously moist and fluffy cake without eggs.

## HOW TO MAKE FLAXSEED AND CHIA "EGGS"

You can also try using a flaxseed or chia "egg". This works well if you don't want added flavour or sweetness as it has a neutral flavour and, when water is added, has a gloopy consistency like egg white. For cakes, grind flax seeds until powdered or use chia seeds whole, then mix 1 tablespoon seeds with 3 tablespoons water to make a batter and leave to sit until thickened. Flax or chia "eggs" also work well in chocolate brownies, gluten-free baking and to help bind pastry.

## MERINGUES AND MARSHMALLOWS

If you want to make meringues, marshmallows, macarons, mousse or even mayonnaise, conventional recipes use whipped egg whites to give that light, fluffy texture. This is where you can use the lightness of whipped aquafaba instead.

Aquafaba is the thick liquid that you usually drain off from a can or jar of chickpeas (or any beans), but amazingly it has a protein structure that works similarly to egg white. You should always use the aquafaba from cans or jars of beans that are water only with no added salt or sugar, and ideally from organic beans, as I find the aquafaba is better from organic brands. The liquid from other beans such as butterbeans (lima beans) and cannellini beans will also work – white beans have the least "beany" colour and flavour.

For meringues, simply whisk the aquafaba liquid with a drop of lemon juice. Use an electric whisk for 5 minutes to form soft peaks, then add equal amounts of sugar, spoon by spoon, whisking well between each addition. It can take a bit longer for aquafaba to thicken up than egg whites – so don't give up too soon.

Aquafaba meringues are usually more fragile than traditional meringues, so you'll need steady hands for making pavlova and they may be too delicate to achieve a perfectly neat finish on a roulade – but the flavour will still be delicious.

## BINDING SAVOURY RECIPES

Eggs are also used in recipes for binding ingredients together. Gram (besan) flour can work well in savoury recipes like burgers and fritters instead of egg. Gram flour does have a slightly odd metallic taste when it's raw, but once it's cooked it disappears completely.

## TARTS, TORTILLA AND QUICHES

These often use eggs both in the pastry and to set the filling, but it's perfectly possible to make both without eggs. A simple pastry can be made with just flour, vegan margarine, salt and water – or try rye flour, which binds even more easily with water with no need for egg.

For the filling, a gram flour batter sets firm with an "eggy" consistency and a neutral taste so it can take up whatever flavour you fancy.

You can also use silken tofu as a substitute in savoury recipes such as quiches. Add 60g (2oz) puréed silken tofu per egg. It's important to keep in mind that although tofu doesn't fluff up like eggs, it does create a texture that's comparable in dishes such as quiche.

## PANCAKES

There are lots of options for replacing eggs in pancakes – using mashed ripe banana with oat or buckwheat flour is popular and these add extra flavour and nutrients to the mix. You can also try using a flaxseed "egg" (see page 167) or switch your usual white flour pancake recipe for socca pancakes, made with gram (besan) flour.

## A SIMPLE GREEN PANCAKE

For a simple green pancake, blitz 150g (5oz) gram flour with 75g (2½oz) spinach leaves, a handful of herbs (try flat-leaf parsley, basil or coriander/cilantro) and some seasoning in a blender with 250ml (8½fl oz) water to make a batter. Heat a little olive oil in a frying pan (skillet), then thinly pour in the batter and cook as you would conventional pancakes. These can be used hot as an omelette alternative and folded over sautéed veg, such as garlicky mushrooms, for a tasty brunch, or use cooled as a wrap with hummus, tomatoes and salad greens. They will keep for a few days in the fridge.

## SCRAMBLED "EGG"

This is not chickpea-based, but is worth noting here while we're on the subject of egg replacements – scrambled tofu makes a pretty decent alternative to scrambled egg. Sauté a finely sliced spring onion (scallion) in a pan until soft, then add some crushed garlic, and ½ teaspoon each of spices such as turmeric (for colour), sweet smoked paprika and cumin. Fry for a minute, then crumble a block of firm tofu into the pan (keeping it fairly chunky) and cook for a few minutes. Pile onto wholegrain toast and top with pan-fried or roasted cherry tomatoes and mushrooms. Finish with a scattering of finely chopped flat-leaf parsley.

## "EGG" SALAD

I first tasted kala namak salt – a type of Himalayan black salt – in Zürich, at the plant-based restaurant chain Tibits (highly recommended if you are ever in Switzerland). I tried their vegan "egg" salad and could hardly believe it wasn't real egg. The secret is the sulphur compounds in the kala namak salt.

To make your own vegan "egg mayo" sandwich, mix a couple of tablespoons of plant-based mayonnaise with a dash of Dijon mustard, a splash of lemon juice and a pinch of turmeric (to add the authentic colour). Season with freshly ground black pepper and a healthy pinch of kala namak and mix in some thinly sliced spring onions (scallions) and a couple of slices of firm tofu cut into small cubes (pat dry before slicing). Taste to check the seasoning and eggy flavour is right, then spread the mixture onto wholegrain bread and top with a strong-flavoured green salad leaf, such as rocket (arugula) or watercress.

## SIGNPOSTS

For more on:
🌱 The benefits of pulses, *see* chapter 8
🌱 The Planetary Health Diet, *see* chapter 2

# CHOCOLATE ORANGE AND TAHINI MOUSSE

*This is a rich chocolate mousse with a velvety texture.
I like to chill it in little espresso cups or tiny jars, and it could
easily be enough for six as it's quite rich, especially if you serve
with a biscuit on the side. Always use a really good quality
chocolate as this is the key flavour – if you use dark or milk
chocolate with a lesser cocoa content, adjust the sugar
quantity down to avoid it being too sweet.*

**Serves 4–6 | Prep time: 25 minutes (+ 1 hour chilling)**

## INGREDIENTS

**200g (7oz) dark
orange chocolate**
(I use a Fairtrade
variety with 70%
cocoa solids)

**80g (3oz) tahini**

**120ml (4fl oz)
aquafaba** (this is
around the amount
of liquid you get from
one 400g/14oz can of
chickpeas/garbanzo
beans or other white
beans)

**100g (31/2oz) caster
(superfine) sugar**

**chopped roasted
hazelnuts**, to serve

## Method

Break the chocolate into small pieces and
place in a metal or glass bowl over a gently
simmering pan of water (ensuring the bowl
and water don't touch to avoid burning
the chocolate). Add the tahini and let the
ingredients melt together until smooth,
stirring frequently. Set aside to cool slightly.

Meanwhile, place the aquafaba and sugar
in a stand mixer (or use a hand mixer) and
whisk for 7–10 minutes until you get stiff
peaks – be patient as this does take a little
longer than it does for egg whites.

Gently fold the slightly cooled chocolate and
tahini mixture into the whipped aquafaba to
preserve the airy texture. Fold through until
thoroughly combined with no streaks.

Pour into small cups, ramekins or jars and
chill in the fridge for at least 1 hour.

Before serving, generously scatter the
tops of the mousses with chopped roasted
hazelnuts.

# 10

# ALL ABOUT
# THE SOY

"Unlike growing public scrutiny on fossil fuel
companies, little public pressure exists to hold
global meat and dairy corporations accountable
for their emissions, even as scientific evidence
mounts that our food system is responsible for up
to 37% of all global emissions."

Institute for Agriculture and Trade Policy, USA[1]

**THE GOAL:**
**TO GRAB A CAPP-OAT-CCINO TO GO**

**R**EMEMBER THE DAYS WHEN THE ONLY NON–DAIRY MILK available at your local coffee shop was soya? Today's dairy alternative market is growing rapidly, and plant milks are made from a wide range of grains, nuts and seeds, most commonly soya, almonds, rice, oats and coconut. But more unusual varieties have also hit the shelves made from ingredients such as cashews, hazelnuts, millet, tiger nuts, spelt, quinoa, chickpeas (garbanzo beans), buckwheat, Brazil nuts, barley, split peas, hemp, flax and peanuts, and they all have different flavours and best uses. It may sound like an obvious point, but you don't have to be vegan to enjoy them; they are a perfectly delicious ingredient choice in their own right, not necessarily a "replacement" for something else. In fact, ordering a cappuccino made with oat or almond milk at your coffee shop is a really good way to give plant milk a try, and you may join the growing number of people who choose plant milks because they prefer the flavour, not necessarily because they are vegan.

Dairy milk is a fairly one-bottle-fits-all product in terms of flavour, and typically your only choice is related to the fat content and creaminess level you prefer or whether it comes from an organic or grass-fed herd. There's so much more choice of flavour with plant milks, and they have different best uses too, as you might prefer one type in your cuppa, but find another is better for baking. Even two milks made with the same basic ingredient – such as almond – from two different brands can have a very different taste and texture. So, if you're not keen on one variety or brand there are plenty more to try, and no doubt more delicious innovations to look forward to as the plant-based milk industry continues to grow.

Delicious as they are, and despite being made from super healthy ingredients, nutritionally plant milks can't always compete with dairy milk, which is naturally high in protein along with other essential vitamins and minerals such as calcium, vitamins D and K and iodine. So, what's the best choice?

"Soya milk is easily the best non-dairy option for protein content; all other non-dairy milks contain very little," says registered nutritionist and author, Anita Bean. "For this reason, plain, unsweetened, calcium-fortified soya milk is the best non-dairy option, especially for children, but it should only be used as a main drink from the age of one (from 6–12 months only breast or infant formula should be given). Bear in mind that soya and other non-dairy milks are also lower in energy than dairy milk, so you'll need to ensure they get enough from other sources. Rice milk should not be given to children under five."

Nut-, grain- and seed-based milks may sound healthy – after all, ingredients such as almonds, oats and flax seeds, are highly nutritious – but as they are usually made with very small amounts of nuts the benefits are similarly small. "Typically, these milks are made with less than 2g nuts per 100ml (3½fl oz) – although a few premium brands contain up to 6g, but that's still tiny. So, the overall nutritional value may be minimal," says Anita. "What you're getting is mainly water, so from a nutritional perspective it's worth ensuring you are eating a good range of whole grains, nuts and seeds in your diet too, which also includes the beneficial fibre."

# NUTRITIOUS QUALITIES OF PLANT MILK

To help you navigate the supermarket aisles, here's an overview of the nutritional hierarchy of plant milks that's worth keeping in mind when you're shopping for an alternative. Whichever type you choose, the healthiest options are unsweetened varieties with no added sugar or other sweeteners.

## 1 FORTIFIED STORE-BOUGHT

We're used to thinking of homemade or organic, additive-free products as the gold standard in food, but plant milks are a rare exception. The best option – at least from a nutritional perspective – is a fortified store-bought product. The reason is that these have added calcium from calcium carbonate (research suggests this form is possibly more easily absorbed by the body[2]) or tricalcium phosphate and often other beneficial nutrients such as vitamin D and iodine, which make them more nutritionally comparable with dairy milk and helpful for replacing the nutrients you may be missing if you're phasing out dairy. Most fortified plant milks contain the same amount of calcium as dairy milk, but as a general rule, look for a milk alternative that contains at least 120mg calcium per 100g. If you're buying soya milk and are concerned about GM soyabeans, look for brands that use non-GM ingredients.

## 2 ORGANIC/NON-FORTIFIED

Organic plant milks are not allowed to be fortified. From an environmental perspective, plant milks made from organic ingredients are going to be a better choice, but an unfortified plant milk is still mostly water and has relatively little nutritional value compared to dairy milk, so make sure you're getting nutrients such as calcium, vitamins D and K, and iodine from other food sources.

## 3 HOMEMADE

Homemade plant milks are very easy to make with nuts or oats, and if you use organic or local ingredients then you'll score eco points too. But even if they contain a higher proportion of the raw ingredients than most commercial varieties, they still don't match up to fortified milk. A homemade milk made using a good value, locally produced product such as oats may be a budget-friendly option if you do a lot of baking. Homemade milks are usually best used on the day you make them and certainly within two days at most, as they don't keep well.

# SHAKE, SHAKE

If you buy a fortified plant milk, always shake it thoroughly before pouring. One study found that you'll only get 30% of the calcium content given on the label from an unshaken drink, so remember the mantra "shake to boost your intake".

In most brands, it's normal for a residue of calcium to be left in the carton so you're unlikely to get 100% of the RDA quoted on the nutritional info panel anyway.

# WHICH PLANT MILK TO CHOOSE?

With so many available, here's a quick overview of the main types of plant milk and their best uses. With so many new brands and types emerging, it's good to try a few to find your favourites.

## SOYA MILK

Higher in protein than other alternatives and containing naturally half the fat of cow's milk, this versatile, creamy milk is probably closest to dairy milk and from a nutritional perspective it's a good all-rounder for a family. Stable at high temperatures, it's reliably good in cooking and baking too.

## ALMOND AND OTHER NUT MILKS

Sweet and nutty, almond milk is made from ground almonds mixed with water but is low in protein compared to soya milk. Thanks to its rich texture and naturally sweet, nutty flavour, it's perfect for breakfasts ranging from chia pudding to porridge, and is also delicious in smoothies, milky desserts and baking. Some like the nutty flavour in coffee too. Overall, almond milk is one of the most popular dairy alternatives. Nutritionally similar to almond, cashew milk is really creamy, so it's great with breakfast cereals but also for making vegan white sauces. Look out for hazelnut milk too, which is higher in fat and calories than other nut milks and makes fantastic hot chocolate and desserts.

## OAT MILK

We all know that oats are good for us, and oat milk offers some of the same nutritional benefits including iron. Made by soaking hulled oats in water, it's low in fat and produces a creamy milk that won't curdle or split when heated like some plant milks, so can be used for making white sauces. If you enjoy a frothy coffee, look for barista varieties, as coffee lovers love foaming oat milks for making authentic cappuccinos.

## RICE MILK

Thinner and more watery than other milks, rice milk is light and non-creamy. If you find soya milk too rich then this might work for you, as it's quite similar to skimmed cow's milk. It's lower in protein and also lower in fat than other plant milks, but it can be fairly sweet, so tends to work better in desserts and for breakfast. It's often too thin to use in baking unless there's another thickening agent in the recipe.

## COCONUT MILK

Coconut milk drinks (not the rich milk from cans) are typically made by soaking the white flesh of coconuts in hot water, then skimming off the cream and using the milk left behind. These drinks are lower in fat than canned coconut milk (typically 2%) and lower in sugar too, but some people still find it tastes quite sweet so use it for making desserts, cakes and smoothies, or in Asian dishes such as Thai and Indian curries.

## BE IODINE AWARE

If you're omitting all dairy products, then you'll need to find alternative sources of iodine. "Dairy milk is a major source of iodine in our diet whereas plant milks contain virtually none," says nutritionist Anita Bean. "We need it for making thyroid hormones and it's also important for growth in young children. Having low levels can lead to a lower metabolic rate and weight gain, and in pregnant women it's linked to lower IQ and reading scores in their children."

There are very few natural sources of iodine in the diet if you don't eat dairy or fortified alternatives. Anita recommends getting your iodine from a multivitamin supplement containing the daily requirement, which is 150 micrograms.

## DO WE NEED TO CUT DAIRY?

From childhood we've been told that milk is good for us, that it grows healthy bones and teeth. But after many years of dutifully eating all my bread crusts, my hair still isn't curly, so is it time to question everything we've been brought up to believe about the healthiness of milk too?

The vegan argument is that cows' milk is the perfect food for calves not humans – one of the hugely successful Swedish oat milk brand Oatly's advertising slogans is: "It's like milk but made for humans" – and many people believe that with so many alternatives available we no longer need to consume dairy milk, especially given its significant contribution to greenhouse gas emissions. While official health advice in most countries is to limit saturated animal fats – such as those contained in full-fat dairy products – a recent Swedish study suggested that dairy products may have a protective effect against heart disease.[3] The point is that research is ongoing and the jury is still out on whether dairy is good for us, but if you're worried you might fall short on your calcium without it, there's no need to panic.

Milk's main claim to fame is that it is rich in calcium, a mineral essential for building strong, healthy bones, which constantly renew and repair throughout our lifetime, and calcium also plays an important role in other functions in the body such as blood clotting and nerve and muscle function. Dairy products do provide a rich and easily digestible source of calcium (for those who don't have lactose malabsorption, at least) and it's in a form that is more easily absorbed by the body than the calcium found in most plant foods. In the post-war years, when milk first started to be heavily promoted as a health food to use up the rivers of excess milk produced thanks to wartime incentives offered to farmers, it made sense to enrich children's diets with this plentiful milk to prevent conditions such as rickets, especially at a time when nutritious food was scarce and alternatives were limited.

But the white stuff is not the only food source of this essential mineral. We need at least 700mg of calcium daily and the good news is that this is relatively easy to achieve even without dairy products. If you add 100g (3½oz or around 4) chopped dried figs to your breakfast and later have a stir fry using 100g (3½oz) tofu, you'll hit your daily calcium target. Just try to be calcium aware at every meal – so if, for example, you choose an unfortified, organic, coconut yoghurt, add some chopped dried figs and sprinkle it with sesame seeds to increase the calcium content.

Boost your intake by including plenty of the following foods, which contain varying levels of calcium.

- Fortified breakfast cereals, such as instant porridge
- Tofu
- Fortified soya yoghurt
- Sesame seeds and tahini (a paste made from sesame seeds)
- Dried and semi-dried figs
- Tempeh
- Bread with added linseed and soya
- White bread (higher in calcium, but wholemeal bread is also a good source and has other benefits)
- Green leafy veg, such as cooked kale, spinach, watercress, pak choi (bok choy), spring greens
- Broccoli
- Nuts and seeds, especially almonds and almond butter, sunflower seeds and chia seeds
- Edamame beans
- Baked beans in tomato sauce

## WHAT'S THE LINK WITH VITAMIN D?

Vitamin D – the sunshine vitamin – plays several roles in our bodies, from helping us absorb calcium from food to promote bone health, to supporting muscle function, the immune system, the brain and nervous system, regulating insulin, lung and cardiovascular health, and may play a role in preventing lifestyle diseases such as some types of cancer, dementia, type-2 diabetes and heart disease. However, studies suggest that up to a third of us could be vitamin-D deficient and have no idea, especially in the winter months, which means you could be making a huge effort to ramp up your plant-based calcium intake, but without sufficient vitamin D it won't be properly absorbed.

Vitamin D is both a hormone – which our bodies make through the action of the ultraviolet light from the sun on our skin – and a fat-soluble vitamin, which is mostly found in foods such as egg yolks and dairy foods, so if you are going completely plant-based then you should include fortified products such as plant milk, plant butter spreads, breakfast cereals and yoghurts in your diet, especially during the winter months. You can also add a handful of mushrooms to your food – if you leave them in a sunny spot for half an hour before eating them, you can boost the vitamin D content.

Currently, the UK Government and NHS guidelines recommend that everyone also takes a daily vitamin D supplement of 10 micrograms (400 International Units) during the autumn and winter months, while the US guidelines recommend 600 IU daily. For better absorption, eat with foods high in healthy fats such as nuts and seeds.

To naturally boost your vitamin D levels, take a daily 15-minute walk in sunlight at around lunchtime when the sun is high in the sky with some of your skin exposed and no sunscreen on – another great reason to make time for a walk every day. If you have darker skin you may need up to 25 minutes or less than 15 minutes if you are very fair.

Also remember that regular weight-bearing and resistance exercise at moderate intensity is also important for maintaining healthy bones.

## GOOD FOR YOU, GOOD FOR THE PLANET

I'm going to level with you – it's not easy to consume milk of any kind in an eco-friendly way. The dairy industry worldwide wields enormous political and commercial clout, and continues to benefit from generous subsidies that encourage substantial over-production, with little regard or regulation for its escalating greenhouse gas emissions. Despite the phenomenal growth of the plant milk industry, production levels of dairy are still soaring in all the major markets such as Europe, the USA, New Zealand and India,

# A NOTE ON ViTAMiN B12

Vitamin B12, often known as folate, is mostly found in meat, fish, eggs and dairy products, so if you're going completely meat- and dairy-free then you may need to take a Vitamin B12 supplement as a back-up to prevent a deficiency that could cause a range of health issues such as anaemia. Ensure you eat plenty of fortified foods, such as cereals or plant milks, while other sources include yeast extract products (such as Marmite) or nutritional yeast flakes. Recommendations for how much B12 we need vary from country to country, but in the UK the Vegan Society suggests aiming to eat fortified foods two or three times a day to get at least 3 micrograms (mcg or µg) of B12 a day, or taking one B12 supplement daily providing at least 10 micrograms or a weekly B12 supplement providing at least 2000 micrograms.

and their emissions increase at a similar rate. A recent report revealed that thirteen of the largest dairy corporations emitted more greenhouse gases than major polluters in the mining and fossil fuel sectors, and combined they had the same emissions as the whole of the UK, the sixth biggest economy in the world.[4]

Studies looking at the $CO_2$ emissions of plant milks produce varying results, because so much depends on where and how the ingredients are grown, the type of ingredients used, along with many other factors. However, on average, a litre of dairy milk produces up to three times as many greenhouse gases as a litre of any type of plant milk, and dairy is the second biggest contributor to greenhouse gas emissions from the food production sector after beef.

Joseph Poore, who led a large review study on $CO_2$ emissions concerning dairy and plant milks in Europe for the University of Oxford, perhaps put it best when asked which plant milk is best for the environment: "I think they're all so low impact compared to dairy milk that if we chose to change to any of them it would generally be beneficial."[5]

That said, it's worth knowing some key facts about some of the leading types of plant milks that have eco and ethical issues associated with their production, to help you make an informed buying choice.

## ALMOND MILK

This is one of the most popular plant milks, but it gets some bad press. Over 80% of the world's almonds are grown in California, and there are concerns that the very thirsty almond monocrop is drinking this already drought-affected state dry. On the other hand, California's dairy industry is far bigger than the almond industry and some figures show it uses more water to grow feed for livestock than it does to grow almonds.

But the massive use of pesticides in almond farming is an even bigger issue, as growers routinely use chemicals that potentially harm human health. These also have devastating effects on pollinator populations, especially on the billions of commercial honeybees brought in specifically to pollinate the almond trees every year, where they are exposed to lethal doses of pesticides such as glyphosate. With a mortality rate of bees far higher than that of all fish and animals raised for slaughter in the US combined,[6] there's a strong argument that almond milk made from Californian nuts can't really be considered either vegan or eco-friendly. The plight of bees has raised awareness of the issue in relation to almond production, but it's worth remembering that all agro-industrial monoculture on this scale has similarly drastic effects on the health of the local ecosystems and beyond.

What to Buy: Look for organic almond milk brands or those that source almonds from other areas, such as Europe.

## COCONUT MILK

Coconut milk – and other products such as coconut water, oil, sugar and flour – have become hugely popular in recent years, in both food and self-care products. But as with many other superfood crops, where farmers in places such as the Philippines, Indonesia and Sri Lanka used to grow coconuts traditionally and sustainably, this is increasingly being replaced with monoculture and all its associated problems. Tree crops like coconut (along with products such as coffee and cacao beans) are often produced by smallholders, many of whom live on the brink of poverty, while their products are bought for low prices and then sold on at a huge premium to wealthier nations.

What to buy: Choose organic coconut products grown without chemicals, which benefits people and planet, and brands certified Fair Trade to ensure smaller producers receive fair prices. Look for independent ethical brands and co-operatives that treat their suppliers well.

## RICE MILK

All grains use a relatively large amount of land to grow in, compared to nut trees. Rice uses a lot of water and emits the most greenhouse gases of the grain crops, thanks to the methane-producing bacteria in flooded rice paddies, although emissions are still substantially less than those produced by the dairy industry. Some rice – and therefore rice milk – contains unacceptably high levels of arsenic (which is why it's not recommended for young children) from synthetic fertilizers used to boost yields, which also pollutes local water supplies and damages ecosystems. Exploitation of low-paid workers is also an issue in rice-growing regions.

**What to buy:** Rice milk is carbon-intensive compared to other plant milks, but if you do buy it then choose organic and Fair Trade brands wherever possible.

## SOYA

This is the tricky one. Soya is controversial, and deforestation in South America caused by soya production has been used as a stick to beat vegans with. But to keep things in perspective, around 75% of the world's soya crop is used for feeding animals – mainly poultry, pigs and farmed fish – with 20% used for soybean oil and only around 5% going directly into human food products.[7]

Despite efforts to halt land being cleared for agriculture in the Brazilian rainforests, with some success thanks to a long-standing "soya moratorium" to prevent crops being grown on freshly deforested land, deforestation for agriculture is still a huge problem. Other contributing factors include changing political leadership, exploitative farmers and companies operating in this industry, and limitations of the moratorium (it doesn't include other important landscapes such as virgin habitat in the neighbouring Brazilian Cerrado, for example) plus loopholes around enforcement.

So, should we avoid eating soya from a sustainability perspective? With 40 million hectares (99 million acres) of land already cleared in Brazil for growing soya, and the fact that a plant-based diet potentially produces around half the emissions of a carnivorous diet, the solution is clear – reducing meat and dairy intake reduces the demand for soya to feed intensively reared animals, which means no further deforestation is needed.

**What to buy**: Try to buy products made with organic, non-Brazilian soya that is as locally produced as possible. Look for brands individually certified by The Roundtable on Responsible Soy and Proterra; and the WWF has produced a helpful soy scorecard at soyscorecard.panda.org.

# PLANT MILKS FOR THE PLANET

When you are choosing a plant milk over dairy, you are already making a choice that has a positive impact on reducing climate change, so feel free to choose a brand based on flavour and price. If you're keen to shop as ethically as possible, look out for independent brands, as some of the leading plant milk products are produced by companies owned by multinational parent companies that also produce dairy produce or engage in other ethically questionable activities.

Less environmentally problematic plant milk choices include oat, hazelnut, hemp, flax, pea, barley and chickpea milk. All of these crops can be grown in cooler climates, which means they don't need vast amounts of additional water and are considered more sustainable if grown in the right way and in the right place. However, where you live in the world also affects any shortlist of "better" plant milks. For example, macadamia nut trees are native to Australia, so macadamia nut milk might be a more eco choice if you live in Sydney.

- **Pea milk** is made from yellow split peas and tastes remarkably similar to dairy milk. Crops such as split peas and chickpeas (garbanzo beans) are nitrogen-fixing, like most beans and pulses, so they promote good soil health.

- **Hazelnut milk** is a better eco choice than almond. The trees are cross-pollinated by wind, which carries dry pollen in the air, so they don't require pollination by bees. They also tend to grow in areas of higher rainfall, so need much less watering. Hazelnuts have not yet become cultivated in a highly intensive way.

- **Hemp seed milk** is fairly new on the scene, mainly due to its close relationship to cannabis. Growing it was legalized in the US in 2018, opening the door for wider use, and it's a highly versatile crop with numerous uses. It's naturally pest- and weed-free, and grows well even in poor soil as it uses little water and nutrients, making it a highly sustainable crop.

- **Barley milk** is tipped to become more popular as this ancient grain is enjoying a renaissance. It's a very sustainable and resilient crop, it can grow almost anywhere in almost any climate and the nutritional benefits are similar to those of oats, including being a source of soluble beta-glucan fibre that helps balance blood cholesterol.

- **Oat milk** can be tricky, as the herbicide glyphosate is often sprayed onto oat crops. Glyphosate is the chemical used in the controversial but widely used weedkiller, Roundup, which has been linked in some scientific studies with cancer. A study by the US Environmental Working Group found that most oat-based foods contained glyphosate, even organic products. In Europe, traces have been found in many foods, including oats, peas, wheat, buckwheat and soya. If you're concerned, choose organic or brands that guarantee their products are glyphosate-free.

# SAY CHEESE, PLEASE

Cheese is one of the most popular products made with milk, and is often the food that people find most difficult to give up. If you need cheese in your life, choose an organic, local variety (farm shops and delis will offer a better variety of ethically produced, artisan cheeses than supermarkets) to savour in small quantities.

If you're ready to dive into the vegan "cheese" market, this is a rapidly evolving sector and there are now some remarkably good plant-based cheese products, including feta-style cubes, melting mozzarella-style slices, grated hard and soft, spreadable "cheese". Usually made from ingredients such as nuts, soya/tofu or coconut oil, and often with some fermenting involved (as in "real" cheesemaking), you'll need to try a few brands because they vary widely in quality and flavour – just don't expect any of them to taste exactly like dairy cheese. Alternatively, nut cheeses are surprisingly simple to master at home with just a few ingredients.

Cashews are often used to produce some cheese replacement products in the kitchen, especially creamy sauces. Or a sprinkle of fortified nutritional yeast adds a savoury Parmesan-ish flavour to dishes – and a good dose of vitamin B12 that is often lacking in vegan diets.

Sometimes it's that unique umami flavour that's missing when you stop using cheese, so try to add it in other ways – fermented ingredients such as miso paste, vegan kimchi and soya sauce or tamari are naturally rich in umami, but toasted nuts and seeds, spices, herbs, chilli and dried seaweed are brilliant flavour enhancers too.

# CASHEW CREAM

*Cashew cream is a versatile dairy alternative that can be used as a dip, a creamy pasta sauce, dolloped onto a bean chilli or even to replace a traditional béchamel sauce. Depending on how you want to use it, you can add fresh herbs, garlic, spices, chilli sauce or nutritional yeast (for a cheesy flavour). For a sweet cream, omit the lemon and salt, and blend in maple syrup, vanilla paste or a couple of soaked dates.*

**Serves 2–4, depending on how you use it**
**Prep time: 5 minutes (+ overnight soaking)**

## INGREDIENTS

**150g (5oz) raw cashews**

**120ml (4fl oz) water**

**1 tablespoon lemon juice**
(optional)

**½ teaspoon sea salt**
(optional)

## METHOD

Soak the cashews in cold water, ideally overnight. You can omit this step if you have a high-speed blender, but it helps to get a creamier result.

Drain the cashews. Put all the ingredients in the blender and blitz. Let the blender run for a while and periodically scrape the sides until you get a super-smooth, velvety texture.

This will keep for around 1 week in the fridge or it can be frozen. Defrost overnight in the fridge.

## HOMEMADE ALMOND MILK

*This is so quick and easy to make – and you can use ethically sourced almonds too. Don't waste the leftover pulp – add it to porridge, smoothies, creamy sauces or use in baking.*

**Serves 2 | Prep time: 5 minutes (+ overnight soaking)**

**INGREDIENTS**

**100g (3½oz) almonds** (ideally organic)

**400ml (13fl oz) water**

**pinch of salt** (optional)

**METHOD**

Place the almonds in a bowl and soak in cold water overnight.

Drain and rinse the nuts, then tip into a blender along with the measured water (for best results, use a high-powered machine, although a standard blender will still work). Blitz until completely blended.

Strain the liquid through a muslin cloth or nut milk bag, decant into a bottle and store in the fridge for no more than 2–3 days.

## SIGNPOSTS

For more on:

🌱 **Ethical plant ingredients,** *see* **chapters 10 and 11**

🌱 **Organic and regenerative food,** *see* **chapter 11**

# 11

# WHY THROW FOOD (AND MONEY) IN THE BIN?

*"If global food waste were a country, it would be the third largest emitter of greenhouse gases after china and the US."*

The Food and Agriculture Organization of the United Nations

**THE GOAL:**
**TO WORK TOWARD A ZERO-WASTE KITCHEN**

**F**ROM A YOUNG AGE MY MOTHER WAS TOLD THAT YOU weren't supposed to eat the stem end of a cucumber because it was poisonous; instead, it had to be sliced off at the point where the seeds start. She continued to do this in her own kitchen and for many years I also routinely chopped a large chunk off the end of my cucumbers. When I started learning more about food waste, I began to question a lot of my ingrained kitchen habits, including our family cucumber trimming tradition. Strangely, I discovered that it didn't originate from an old wives' tale, as I expected, but from the fact that the stem end of the cucumber used to be the bitterest part – caused by a concentration of a toxic compound called cucurbitacin – so there was some basis for the superstition that the end of the cucumber was poisonous. However, over generations, the bitterness has been bred out of the traditional English cucumber, so no trimming is required, except for the tiny hard stem.

Many of us have quite a few entrenched habits like this. We may always peel butternut squash before cooking, or routinely strip away the outer leaves of a round lettuce, or cut off and discard the leafy tops of carrots or beetroot. But we need to rethink these habits, because we are wasting up to 30% of our fresh produce through needless trimming and peeling, and this is wasteful in three respects – firstly it's throwing away perfectly edible produce and contributing to a huge global food waste problem; secondly, it's a tremendous loss of valuable nutrition that could improve our wellbeing; and finally, it's throwing our hard-earned money in the bin.

It has taken me years to realize a simple fact – wholefoods and whole foods are the same thing. I know, it sounds obvious when I see it written like this, and apologies if you've already made this mental leap but honestly, I think a lot of us don't see the connection as clearly as we should. Let me explain. The ideal of living plantfully is to adopt a predominantly wholefood, plant-focused diet, and this means eating foods in their natural state and valuing every edible part of them. For example, choosing brown rice or wholemeal flour with the bran and germ of the grains retained – along with all their nourishing vitamins, minerals, antioxidants and fibre – instead of refined white rice or white flour, which have had all this goodness removed.

But I've also come to realize that following a wholefood diet doesn't just mean choosing products that have been minimally processed by a farmer, producer or manufacturer, it also refers to what WE do to that food when it arrives in our kitchen. It means valuing and eating the whole food wherever possible, whether that's cauliflower leaves, herb stems, potato skins or pumpkin seeds, which all contain nutrients that are hugely beneficial for our health. Most of us don't get nearly enough fibre, and this is partly because we eat too many refined and processed products and not enough whole fruit, veg and other plant foods, and also because we routinely throw away the parts of food that contain the most fibre such as peels and skins.

Different bits of fruit and vegetables offer different health benefits to the "main" ingredient, and may even be cooked or used in a different way. So, for example, the more commonly used root part of beetroot (beets) is rich in heart-friendly nitrates and betacyanin, which gives the beetroot its purple colour and has antioxidant properties thought to help suppress some kinds of cancer, to name just a couple of benefits. But the greens, which are usually chopped off before they reach the supermarket, are even more nutritious than kale, and are also packed with essential nutrients, antioxidants and fibre. Beetroots are typically boiled or oven roasted, while the leaves might be eaten raw, steamed or stir-fried, making this one vegetable incredibly versatile in the kitchen.

Many of the odds and ends we routinely throw away are not foods that we've accidentally let go beyond their date or that have gone dry, limp or mouldy, but perfectly fresh and edible bits we deliberately remove from fruit and vegetables out of habit or convention. This might also include wonky, raggedy or less-than-perfect looking fruit and veg, which still have all the flavour and nutrients of supermarket-standard produce – possibly even more if they are home or organically grown. These could all be transformed into delicious food, with just a little creativity and know-how.

Sourcing produce from places that enable you to use the whole vegetable, whether that means growing your own, shopping at a farmers' market or using an organic veg box delivery, means you enjoy all these "extra" ingredients. By challenging our ingrained trimming practices, we not only start to make a difference to food waste, we also have an opportunity to improve our health and wellbeing by eating every last nutritious bit of the produce we buy. And the best bit? Managing your kitchen in this thrifty way – just like our grandmothers did – means you'll end up saving a lot of money too.

# GOOD FOR YOU, GOOD FOR THE PLANET

"There's a huge waste of nutrition that occurs when we don't use whole foods," agrees Tom Hunt, a pioneering zero-waste chef, food writer and author of sustainable manifesto-meets-cookbook *Eating for Pleasure, People and Planet.*[1] "I recommend you buy the best food you can afford, which doesn't have to be organic if that's not in your budget, but by eating every last scrap of the fruit and veg you buy, you can make savings and create a surplus to spend on better quality food," he says. "If you are saving 20–30% of your expenditure on food because you're eating the 20–30% you previously would have wasted, that represents the typical extra cost of organic products. This means it can work out as cost neutral to eat a predominantly wholefood, plant-rich diet that includes organic produce, while also reducing your waste. Remember that anything you're able to spend on improving your diet is an investment in your own health and that of your family and community."

Tom's brilliant philosophy of "Root to Fruit Eating" has three core principles: eat for pleasure, eat whole foods and eat the best food you can. It's all about placing a higher value on your food in every respect – from enjoying what you eat as a route to improving your own health; basing your diet on nutritious wholefoods – and using every bit of them to save money and reduce waste; and investing in the best quality ingredients you can afford, ideally produced in an organic or regenerative way, which benefits you, your local community and the planet.

"The main reason we waste food is because it has lost its true value," says Tom. "We've lost touch with the origins of our food and the clear answer is to try and mend those connections. We all need to engage with our food – where it comes from, how it is grown – and this can be both an enjoyable and enlightening process.

"If we accept the notion that food is nature ingested, then by reconnecting with food we are reconnecting with nature. Root to Fruit Eating is a way to not only heal our broken food system but also to heal our own health and that of the environment."

## THE CLIMATE CONNECTION

So, how exactly does throwing away cauliflower leaves or a pack of squishy tomatoes contribute to global warming? The link is more direct than you might expect. Global food waste alone is responsible for 8–10% of all greenhouse gas emissions, and recent research from WRAP, the UK-based environmental charity focused on improving resource efficiency, suggests that while the majority of people say they are concerned about climate change, only around a third of them have made the crucial connection between food waste and its environmental impact.[2]

"People seem much more able to make the link between issues such as plastic pollution and the impact on the planet than between food waste and climate change, probably because it's a more mysterious, less visible connection," says Helen White, special advisor on household food waste at WRAP. "One of our campaign messages is 'wasting food feeds climate change' because we want people to know that it isn't just a slice of bread, it isn't just a tomato, it isn't just a potato that goes into the bin. What is wasted is all the resources that have gone into producing that food and getting it onto your plate. We want people to try and visualize the whole journey of their food and how this enormous set of resources is going to waste when even a small amount is thrown away."

Most of us are now aware that every food product, whether it's bananas, biscuits or beef, has a carbon footprint, and the size of this depends on a variety of factors, including where and how it is produced. Greenhouse gas emissions are associated with every stage of food production, from growing or rearing it – which also includes the use of resources such as water, land use change (potentially including deforestation), production of animal feed and chemical manufacture and use – to processing and packaging. Then there's transportation by land, sea and air; the resources used in retail outlets such as energy for refrigeration; and finally, the fuel used to transport it home by car or delivery van, then refrigerate and cook it. All this is wasted – along with its nutrient potential – when "just a tomato" ends up in the bin.

Food miles make a substantial contribution to a food's carbon footprint. If you have a taste for exotic or global ingredients, they have to be transported long distances, and sometimes everyday foods do too. But not all food miles are equal. Air-freighted food from a closer country may have a bigger climate impact than food exported by sea from the other side of the world, while food produced locally in season will usually have the least impact. For example, while bananas are often imported from tropical regions, they generally travel by sea. Compare that to the relatively huge footprint of soft fruit like strawberries when they are out of season locally, which will either be imported by air from a hotter country or produced locally but in energy-guzzling hothouses.

"The thing is that everyone loves an avocado, don't they?" says Jen Gale, author of *The Sustainable(ish) Living Guide,* "But the impact of air freighted goods is huge. If you're comparing food that's grown locally and in season with something like asparagus flown in from Peru or grapes from South Africa, then you are looking at it potentially having 20 times the impact. It's why we need to think about eating predominantly local and seasonal food as much as possible. We're so used to being able to buy everything all year round we don't even know what's in season, and sometimes we want to eat something more exotic than turnips in winter. It's not a black and white decision – you just have to make the most sensible choices you can that suit your circumstances and budget."

Jen says she'd like to see governments mandating clearer sustainability labelling on food packaging, so people know exactly how far products have travelled and whether it's by land, sea or air, which may also make people think twice about chucking it away uneaten. "Even something as simple as an airplane sticker on air-freighted food would help people make an informed decision about what they are buying," she says. "I have that dilemma in the supermarket regularly. I live in the UK so a typical choice might be between the organic apples from New Zealand or the non-organic from South Africa, which is closer. However, even imported apples have a relatively low carbon footprint as they are usually transported by ship thanks to their long shelf life, so in this case I'd go for the organic option to support better farming practices, if local apples weren't available. But having to make this decision for every type of produce, every time you shop throughout the year, it's not easy."

Put simply, we can lower our carbon footprint substantially simply by basing our diet predominantly on minimally processed food that's grown locally, in season and ideally, organically or regeneratively. And this is true whether you're a carnivore, a vegan or something in between. Not wasting food – along with all the energy and resources that have been expended to get it onto your plate – is one of the easiest ways to reduce your individual impact too.

The attitude that some level of food waste is inevitable and acceptable means that in the UK alone 20 million slices of perfectly edible bread are thrown away every day, which adds up to a million loaves a day[3] – just in one country. When you hear numbers like that, it starts to seem a like bigger deal, doesn't it?

Globally, around a third of all the food produced is lost or wasted, while in 2020 an estimated 9.9% of the world's population suffered from chronic undernourishment (around 800 million people).[4] It's mindboggling. What's fascinating about this issue is that we always come back to the fundamental link between food waste and nutrient waste. When we talk about undernourishment, we often think about famine and poverty, but it's not just a problem for developing countries. We are not only wasting food at every stage from farm to fridge, we are also buying too much and eating too much – of all the wrong things. In countries like the UK and USA, where both good food and heavily processed, often nutritionally valueless, foods are abundant and readily available, there's a crisis of both malnutrition – which also includes over-consumption and its associated lifestyle diseases – and food poverty. And these health issues are wrapped up with a climate impact too. In its 2021 Net Zero report, WRAP suggests that reducing our individual calorie intake to 2500kcal a day could reduce malnutrition while contributing a saving of 6.6 million tonnes of $CO_2e$. The cumulative carbon benefit to achieving the goal of Net Zero by 2050 would be a saving of 135 million tonnes $CO_2e$ – equivalent to taking all the UK's cars and taxis off the road for around two years.[5]

The thing is, unlike many causes of climate change, food waste is something we all have enormous power to influence by making small but significant changes. We live in a global economy and it's unrealistic to think that we're going to only eat exclusively locally grown produce, and we can't have complete control over where all our food is grown – unless you're a self-sufficient smallholder or prepared to be incredibly strict about what you buy. But once food comes home in our shopping bag, we are in complete charge of what happens to it. I think that's a pretty empowering thought at a time when the scale of our environmental challenges feels a little overwhelming.

"After food leaves the farm, it gets wasted through retail, manufacturing, distribution, hospitality and food service, but those combined make up only 30% of food waste," says Helen. "So, 70% is wasted from our own homes. Sometimes I don't think that comes across strongly enough, people don't realize that most UK food waste is household food waste. If we can all better understand the journey of where food comes from and start thinking of it as a precious resource, we are much less likely to waste it."

## MOVING TOWARD A ZERO-WASTE KITCHEN

Do a food waste audit for a week. Write down every bit of food you throw away and be honest – include it on the list if you would normally throw it away – and tot up the approximate value using your last shopping receipt. It's a useful exercise to see just how much food – and cash – you could be wasting in a typical week. It really does make you think twice before throwing even a small portion of food away.

Next time you find something in the cupboards you know you'd never eat, or are hovering over the bin with a packet of something that's slightly past its best, pause. Take a moment to think if it could be rescued. Can it be frozen? Cooked and turned into something else? Donated? Given away through a food sharing app, or a community fridge or food bank? If there's really no other option, could it at least be composted?

The financial savings for your family can be substantial too. In the UK, for example, each household wastes on average the equivalent of eight meals a week, and the total cost of the food that could have been eaten but is thrown away is around £14 billion. That's around £60 per month for the average family with children.[7]

# THE METHANE MOUNTAIN

We already know that sending stuff to landfill is a "bad thing". There is no "away" – so throwing things "away" means they have to be taken elsewhere, whether it's to your local rubbish dump or shipped off to be recycled in other countries, where it often ends up in their landfills or in the ocean. It may be out of sight and out of mind as far as we're concerned, but that stuff is still polluting the planet somewhere.

A plastic bottle may take up to 450 years or more to degrade, leaching toxins into the Earth as it does so, contaminating the ocean with microplastics, causing harm to marine life and finding its way into our soil, water supply and into us too. By contrast, waste food can enrich our soil when turned into compost. Food is organic matter and fully biodegradable; it rots down very quickly with the help of oxygen and bacteria. This might make you think it's not as "bad" to send it to landfill as plastic. However, while food waste can become a beneficial by-product when it's on a properly managed compost heap where the rotting waste remains oxygenated, in landfill, as more junk is piled on top of the junk below, the lower layers become compressed and sink further down the pile, creating the anaerobic (oxygenless) conditions that produce methane. This gas has a global warming potential 21 times greater than carbon dioxide and methane from landfill represents an enormous 40% of the UK's methane output.[7]

Building these brilliant food-saving ideas, including some great tips from Love Food Hate Waste, into your routine will eventually save you time and money.

- **Plan for life.** Meal planning is a great idea – but don't plan ahead for a whole week, especially if you know your life can be unpredictable. Try a two-, three- or four-day plan instead, depending on what works best for your lifestyle. Even if you tend to do a "weekly shop", you don't have to shop for every meal for the whole week, especially if you use your freezer and some of the other time- and food-saving tactics described in this section.

- **Be realistic.** Many of us aspire to cook fresh food from scratch every night, but it doesn't always happen. Accept that plans or your mood may change – just have a plan for what to do with the food that is now at risk of going to waste because you ordered a takeaway, whether that's popping it in the freezer or cooking it anyway to eat tomorrow.

- **Take a shelfie.** Food waste advice usually begins with "write a shopping list", but honestly, is there anything duller than laboriously writing everything out? It just feels like doing homework. Instead, Helen suggests taking a photo of your fridge, food cupboard and even freezer drawers before you go shopping. If you have a meal plan in mind and shelfie pics on your phone, that's all you need. If you like a list, then try a "running" list for the regular stuff that might not be on your meal plan like tea bags or juice – keep a list in the notes section on your phone (or a dedicated app), and every time you finish a packet of something, add it to the list there and then, before you forget.

- **Go online.** Use modern technology to your advantage. Some people may find that online shopping prevents overbuying as it's easier to create a list of favourites, avoid impulse purchases and your fridge and cupboards are right there to check as you shop. However, don't fall into the trap of buying the same things on autopilot every week, as this leads to waste.

- **Cook it.** If you've got a box of mushrooms that look a bit dry or a pack of veggie sausages on the use-by date, cooking them gives you a couple more days to eat them and once cooked, it's even quicker to make them into a meal.

- **Make a dish for later.** If you've got some veg that's looking a bit past its best, turn it into something else. A tray of roasted vegetables, a smoothie, a pasta sauce, a soup are all great options for extending the life of fresh produce, and many can be frozen too.

- **Don't cook too much.** This is about clever portion control as over-portioning leads to waste –and expanding waistlines! Helen suggests a great portioning tip here. "One standard coffee mug of dried rice filled to the brim is enough to feed four people. If you do cook too much, just cool it quickly and either freeze or put it in the fridge and use it within 24 hours, reheated thoroughly. Get an eye for portion sizes of foods such as grains and pasta that work for your family or get in the habit of weighing them (for example, 75g/2½oz is considered to be one portion of uncooked pasta), and be savvy about how much you use in the first place." Excess cooked pasta can be stored in the fridge or freezer and revived by reheating in boiling water for a few minutes.

- **Always cook too much.** This time we are talking about batch cooking. This doesn't mean spending the whole of Sunday in your apron sweating over huge veggie lasagnes and lentil cottage pies, unless you want to, of course. It can just mean cooking for four every time you cook for two. Serve up two portions of today's meal and stash two in the fridge or freezer for another day.

- **Reinventing leftovers.** "Leftovers need an image makeover," says Helen. "The name suggests something second-hand and not that appetizing, but leftovers can be the basis of an amazing new meal." For example, I like to make a big tray of roasted vegetables with harissa, fresh thyme, garlic and pre-cooked lentils: on the first day I'll serve it with steamed greens, and the next as a baked potato topping with a dollop of plant-based tahini yoghurt or hummus.

When you combine leftovers from the fridge or freezer with a few storecupboard staples or some extra fresh veg, it becomes a different dish, so you don't have to eat the same meal twice.

- **Shop from your cupboards.** For one week a month, challenge yourself to avoid going shopping, except for a few fresh basics, and use up the food you already have in the kitchen. When I do this, I'm always amazed by the variety of meals I can produce without buying any extra food.

- **Understand best-before dates.** While use-by dates are a hard deadline printed on higher-risk foods such as meat and dairy for safety reasons, best-before dates are a guide to quality. If it's gone beyond the best-before date, use your common sense to decide if it's still good to eat.

- **Get it delivered.** A weekly organic veg box is a great investment in better farming, better quality food and it helps you try new ingredients and stay connected with seasonal eating too.

- **Store it safely.** It may sound obvious, but correct storage significantly prolongs the life of food. Check the best places to keep different products – for example, many people put oranges and lemons in a fruit bowl, but they are best kept in the fridge. Use clips to properly seal bread bags and dry food packets, and although Tupperware containers are plastic, they can be reused endlessly to store leftovers. The plastic or foil containers from the takeaway can be washed out and re-used for freezing individual portions of meals. It's best to avoid single-use clingfilm (saran wrap) but there's no need for expensive beeswax wraps (nice as they are) – just popping a plate over a bowl will keep food fresh.

For more ideas, Lovefoodhatewaste.com has loads of brilliant suggestions for repurposing food, correct storage advice for all types of produce and many more tips and tricks.

# GET FREEZER SAVVY

There are very few foods you can't freeze, except tender veg with a high water content, such as salad leaves and cucumber. Plant and dairy milk, egg whites, chopped onions, pulses, tofu, even wine, can be safely frozen. There's a useful A-Z of Food Storage at lovefoodhatewaste.com.

- You can freeze right up to the use-by date, and this enables you to "press pause" and buy more time to eat the food.

- Try to keep a bit of space free in the freezer specifically to store spare food and leftovers, as this is also a good tactic for making easy meals another day.

- Freeze in single portion sizes so you don't end up having to defrost a whole "mealberg" when you only need one portion.

- Don't let your freezer become a mortuary for food, only delaying its exit to the bin. Find realistic solutions for leftover food and only freeze things you know you will actually use.

- If you know you have a habit of wasting fresh produce, buy more frozen or canned vegetables and fruit. Studies show that many kinds of frozen produce are just as nutritious as fresh, if not more, including highly perishable fruits such as berries, and vegetables such as peas and sweetcorn that are frozen very soon after harvesting to preserve their goodness.

# 10 BRILLIANT REPURPOSING IDEAS

To prove almost everything can be salvaged, here are a few suggestions for using up leftovers or those leaves and stems that often get discarded.

Remember, it's good practice to always wash your fruit and veg before use, but it's especially important to remove any surface chemical residues if you're using peels, skins and outer leaves of non-organic produce.

## 1 SOUR MILK

Not so great on cereal, but perfect for making light and fluffy scones. Make savoury scones with fresh herbs to go with soup, which can be frozen and defrosted individually when needed.

## 2 STALE BREAD

Sprinkle stale loaves with water and refresh in the oven, or make croutons for soup or salad by cutting into cubes, sprinkling with oil and baking on a lowish heat until golden and crisp.

Whizz into breadcrumbs and make gratin toppings for roasted veggies with garlic and herbs (*see* page 139). Tear and add to Italian panzanella salad or to sauces and soup as a thickener.

## 3 POTATO AND OTHER ROOT VEG PEELINGS

Drizzle scrubbed peels with olive oil and herbs such as rosemary or thyme, or spices such as paprika, season and bake to make homemade "crisps" for snacks or to top dishes.

## 4 MASHED POTATO

Mix the mash with flour to make gnocchi and serve with broccoli pesto (*see* opposite).

Mash can also be combined with stir-fried onions, shredded greens such as kale, Brussels sprouts and cabbage, and seasoning, and fried in the pan to make "bubble and squeak" fritters.

## 5 TOMATOES

Can be frozen whole and then added straight to dishes such as curries or pasta sauce instead of using canned tomatoes.

Cherry tomatoes on the brink of over-squishiness are great roasted with olive oil, chickpeas (garbanzos) or cannellini beans, garlic, fresh thyme and seasoning. Serve with some good bread, whizz up into a quick soup with some added stock or pile onto pasta.

## 6 BROCCOLI STEMS

These can be finely chopped and steamed with the broccoli florets, or used for pesto.

Roast the whole broccoli with a little oil and seasoning in the oven for about 20–25 minutes until softened and the florets are starting to colour. Whizz the roasted broccoli stem in a food processor with a glug of extra virgin olive oil, a handful of walnuts, a crushed garlic clove, a handful of basil leaves and stems and the juice of ½ lemon. Taste – season if necessary – and serve with a grain, pasta or gnocchi, topped with the roasted broccoli florets.

## 7 CAULIFLOWER LEAVES

If you're making a gratin or cauliflower cheese, add the shredded leaves too for extra flavour and goodness; cauliflower greens can be treated like any other green veg: simply stir-fry in a little oil with some aromatics such as chilli or garlic, season and serve.

Or toss in oil, salt and pepper, and roast in the oven for 5–10 minutes – they go deliciously crispy. It's usually best to trim the very woody end off the base of the stems.

## 8 HERB STEMS

The stems of soft herbs such as basil, parsley and coriander (cilantro) are just as nutritious and delicious as the leaves. They can be added to blended sauces such as pesto, or chopped finely and added to salsa verde, salsa, salads, vegetable stock, soups (add close to the end of cooking) or falafel.

## 9 SOFT FRUITS

These expensive berries spoil quickly. Make a quick fruit chia jam with squishy berries by cooking in a saucepan with chia seeds, maple or agave syrup and vanilla bean paste until the fruit is broken down and the jam has thickened.

Use for desserts, pancakes, yoghurt or cereal. Add berries to muffins, simply purée and freeze in ice-cube trays and add to smoothies or melt in a pan with a little sugar or syrup for a quick fruit sauce.

## 10 LEMON PEEL

Once squeezed, there are plenty of ways to use citrus rinds. You can freeze them and use as zest for baking; cut them into strips, bake in the oven and dry them (or leave pith-side up on a sunny windowsill for a few days) and store in an airtight jar to add to fruit loaf or herbal tea.

Make lemon-zest sugar, lemon-infused vinegar for dressings or lemon-rind marmalade, or add rinds to your homemade cleaning products (*see* page 250).

## SIGNPOSTS

**For more on:**

🌱 Gut health, *see* chapters 3 and 7

🌱 Using herbs, *see* chapter 4

🌱 Organic and regenerative food, *see* chapter 10

🌱 Composting, *see* chapter 3

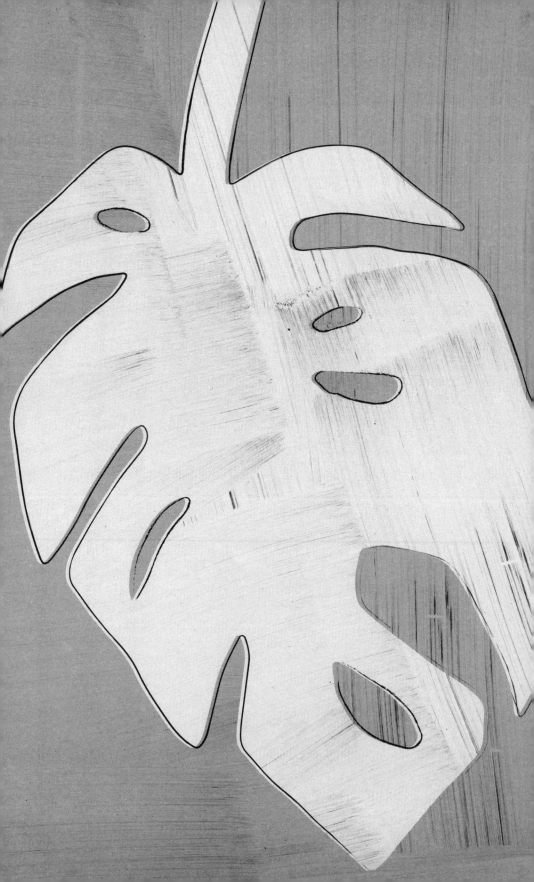

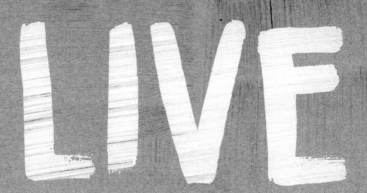

# LIVE

When you start living plantfully through growing and cooking, you'll naturally become more aware of how plants can enhance every aspect of your life. Foraging encourages you to take a closer look at weeds, shrubs and trees you may previously have walked straight past, enabling you to tune into the smallest miracles taking place in the natural world around you – and you may even find delicious things to eat too. Plants have long been foraged and cultivated for their healing properties, and you can use these potent powers to create a nourishing self-care ritual that makes you look as good on the outside as you feel on the inside. You'll also benefit from a more mindful approach to caring for your home through using natural cleaning products and harnessing the healing powers of house plants.

# 12

# CELEBRATING WEEDS AND WILD THINGS

"weeds are flowers too, once you get to know them."

A.A. Milne

**THE GOAL:**
**TO GO FORAGING FOR FUN – AND FOOD**

**G**ROWING UP, WE OFTEN TOOK A BASKET TO THE WILDER EDGES of the village, where we picked fruits and flowers from hedgerow and field, returning home with an abundant haul of blackberries, rosehips or dandelions, whatever was in season at the time. Much of this bounty was destined for Dad's homemade wine, which bubbled away mysteriously in the kitchen for weeks, fizzing with an earthy, sweet-sour aroma that made me think I would never drink wine if the smell was any clue to the final flavour. As a fringe benefit, we enjoyed blackberry and apple crumble and rosehip syrup drizzled on rice pudding. Back then, we didn't call it "foraging", we were just children with an ice-cream tub to fill, enjoying the hunt for wild treasures, and we didn't have to go far to find incredible riches.

The fact that food is growing wild out there – all kinds of edible produce that we didn't plant and don't control – shouldn't be that surprising. Before farming got underway around 10,000 years ago, our hunter-gatherer ancestors were adept at knowing where and in what season to find tubers, leaves, shoots, roots and berries that were delicious, safe to eat and provided an important source of nutrition.

These days, when almost all the food we eat is intensively cultivated and some is so processed it barely resembles anything our ancestors would recognize as food at all, foraging has become an exciting way to reconnect with nature and tap into our primal delight in making a wild edible discovery. It's a wonderful way for those who can't or don't want to grow their own vegetables, or who don't have a garden to grow in, to still enjoy a relationship with nature and the bounty it offers in each season.

Looking to the future, food security may become an issue as our climate changes, and there's comfort in knowing that there is food out there if we only know where to look for it.

## INTO THE WILD

Foraging is easy and anyone can do it. You don't have to be an expert or trek for miles into the wilderness to find things that taste good, have healing properties or nutritional superpowers, because beneficial plants grow absolutely everywhere. The plants that are the most useful to us are often the most common and familiar species, growing in plain view close to where we live. It's almost as if nature designed it that way.

The wild is open to all, and most fruits and nuts such as blackberries or crab apples need no specialist skills or knowledge to forage – just a keen eye and a willingness to try something new. Many of us probably remember foraging as children, but later feel a little self-conscious about doing it or unsure of what to make with our finds. But in the days of taking "bags for life" everywhere we go, and the vast resources of online advice and recipes available to us, we are always ready for foraging.

The best way to start is to choose something you recognize that grows near you, and see how it changes through the seasons. Understand where the plant grows, how it looks at different times of the year, how it evolves in flavour and how to use different parts of it. When you start doing this, it's amazing how your faculties of looking, learning and really seeing something start to develop, and it makes foraging a much richer experience. Plants can change in appearance and edibility throughout the year as they progress from shoots to leaves to flowers and fruit, and they may have different uses or taste better – or become less pleasant or even harmful to eat – in different seasons.

It can feel intimidating to open a field guide and find a mass of Latin names and unfamiliar terminology, complicated advice on how and when to pick, and warnings that some delicious species may be visually similar to other highly poisonous varieties. But don't let this put you off. With time and experience, you'll soon be skillfully spotting and picking more unusual varieties too.

On a guided foraging expedition in the Brecon Beacons, I met expert forager and author of *The Hedgerow Handbook,* Adele Nozedar, who agrees it's best to take it slow. "Almost every plant has some kind of medicinal or edible use for humans in one way or another, and if you tried to learn about all of them at once it would be overwhelming."

While it's thrilling to return home with a basket brimming with good things to eat, foraging is about so much more than eating your finds. "If we want to make the world a better place, and we want to feel we are connected to nature, then going out and looking for plants, picking plants and understanding them is really important – it's an education we all need," says Adele.

"It's important to learn about plants that are not edible too, as they are still vital in our ecosystem. Sometimes people refer to plants that are poisonous as 'evil', but they are not evil; they might not be obviously useful to human beings, but plants are not just here for our benefit, and the more you go foraging, the more you understand this."

A brilliant example is the yew tree. Highly toxic to humans and most animals, eating just a few leaves could make you very ill and may even be fatal. For this reason, yew has become a symbol of death and doom over the centuries, and these ancient trees are often found in church graveyards – although probably mostly to ensure farmers didn't allow livestock to graze there rather than for any mystical purpose. However, the same taxane alkaloids in yew that make it highly poisonous have been used to develop very effective chemotherapy drugs.[1]

The possibility that cures for life-limiting human diseases may be disappearing forever along with the species that contain them when they become extinct is just one powerful reason why preserving biodiversity is so vital for our survival. The ground-breaking American biologist Edward O Wilson makes this clear in his important work, *The Diversity of Life*, by reminding us that we can't put a true value on biodiversity because it's impossible to fully understand the value of each species to future generations. If, as he says, we have already lost 99% of all the species that have ever lived on Earth, who knows what potential cures may have already disappeared with them?

"The medicinal qualities of plants can be quite mysterious," says Adele. "So many drugs and medicines were originally engendered in the natural world from plants. There may be many more potential cures hidden in plants just waiting for us to find, which is another reason why it's terribly important that we don't allow any species to go extinct.

"There is so much more to foraging than just going on an outing or finding food. As your knowledge grows, it becomes a deeply philosophical experience that enables you to connect with the rhythms of the natural world."

# DO NO HARM —
# HOW TO FORAGE SUSTAINABLY

Many edible plants grow in abundance, but still need to be picked with care and in modest quantities to avoid waste, to leave plenty for wildlife and to allow the plant to reproduce for next year.

Wild garlic, for example, tends to grow generously in lush drifts in sunlight-dappled woodland areas, but it's important to only take the leaves and not pull up the bulbs. Unlike the bulbs of garlic we normally buy or grow, only the young leaves, flowers and immature seed pods of wild garlic should be harvested.

Some species have become increasingly rare due to habitat loss, so it's important to avoid picking anything that is endangered – or in danger of becoming so. Edible flowers in decline in the wild, such as cowslips and lady's smock, are best left for the bees, butterflies and other pollinators to enjoy, even though many books about foraging do include them and even suggest recipes.

In the southwest of England, there's a village not far from where I live that is home to the very rare Bath asparagus (also known as Spiked Star of Bethlehem), and in recent years villagers have had to keep watch to deter unwelcome foragers who sometimes uproot the bulbs as they pick to sell the slender stems to upmarket restaurants. It's more than bad manners to be so careless – this rare species takes five years to flower and irresponsible foraging may mean there's nothing to harvest in future years and ultimately may lead to the loss of the entire species.

# POOR MAN'S SPINACH

For every rare species, there are many others in plentiful supply. Everyone will recognize the common nettle (*Urtica dioica*), one of the most ubiquitous plants on the planet. It's also a nutritional powerhouse that is so good for us that the Romans made a point of taking nettles with them when they went a-conquering to ensure they'd have a regular supply wherever they landed. The ancient Greeks were fans too, and "urtication" became established in folklore over the centuries as a remedy for conditions such as arthritis, rheumatism and even paralysis. In 1729, the Scottish physician William Buchan detailed the treatment of palsy in his domestic medicine textbook, published in 1779, reporting that "Some pretend to have found great benefit from rubbing the affected parts with nettles".[2]

You might wince when you read this supposed "cure", because nettles are not only highly skilled at thriving in almost any conditions, they also have an efficient built-in deterrent to hungry animals or foragers: fine hairs that deliver a painful sting caused by formic acid if you so much as accidentally brush a bare leg against a leaf on a walk. The idea of flagellating your limbs with nettles probably doesn't sound very appealing, and for many, picking these feisty plants may not seem worth the effort either.

According to Scottish legend, for nettles to have medicinal value as a tonic, they had to be "unspoken" – which meant being picked at midnight and no one could speak to the gatherer or the medicine wouldn't be effective. If you'd like to go out nettle picking at midnight, then by all means try it, but if you're picking to enjoy the flavour and nutrition of nettles, head out in daylight and keep these tips in mind:

- Prepare as if for battle – wear sturdy footwear, cover arms and legs and use thick gardening or rubber gloves at the very least. Remember though, once picked, wilted nettles lose their sting and can be safely handled in the kitchen.

- Pick while the plants are young, typically in spring while the nettles are no more than knee-high and the leaves are at their freshest. By the time the nettle's droopy flower heads emerge in late spring/early summer, the flavour becomes less palatable, the texture coarsens and becomes gritty and they may even cause stomach upsets. However, nettles that are cut back may also show fresh regrowth in late summer and early autumn (fall), so you can enjoy picking the young leaves again at this time.

- As with all foraging, aim to pick in areas away from traffic pollution, which are unlikely to have been sprayed with herbicides by the local council and are not too close to footpaths where "dog vinaigrette" may have tainted the crop.

- To pick, cut the stem off at the top of the nettle to get around 10–12 young leaves. Lay out your picked nettles on a tray to wilt and the sting will be deactivated – you can then safely strip the leaves from the stems.

- Don't be tempted to sample a raw leaf, even after wilting – nettles must always be cooked before eating.

After braving the sting, is the prize worth it? Nettles have a mild, earthy flavour, and some people find the texture more pleasant than kale. The nutritional benefits are even greater. If you have favourite recipes that call for spinach or kale (anything except salads), cooked nettles can be used instead of, or in combination with, these leafy vegetables, so try them in frittata, soup, fritters, risotto, stir-fries, pasta sauce, herbal tea or on a pizza.

Nettles can go a bit sludge-coloured when cooked and nettle tea can be on the murky, earthy side – let's just say it looks and smells like it's good for you – but I promise it tastes delicious. I like to add herbs such as mint or lemon verbena to lift the fragrance and flavour of a nettle brew.

Expert forager and author John Wright offers a good nettle cooking tip: "Cooked briefly in hot water, blanched in cold water and puréed, it has endless uses, my favourite being for a risotto. Blanching, incidentally, retains the bright green colour; without it the nettles turn an unappetizing brown."[3]

You might wonder why you should bother to gather nettles, when bags of spinach and kale can be bought without peril of pain in the supermarket? Consider though, that nettles come with no legacy of plastic packaging, intensive energy use, added chemicals or food miles like many cultivated greens, and they grow so abundantly that picking them won't cause a conservation issue. Plus, nettles are both free and highly nutritious.

## NUTRITIONAL NOTES

There's really no sting in the tail from nettle picking, because these greens are incredibly nourishing. Packed with vitamins A, C, K and several Bs too, they also contain healthy fats, a complete set of essential amino acids and a generous dose of antioxidant polyphenols, which among many other benefits, help to reduce inflammation. However, pregnant women should avoid nettles as they may trigger uterine contractions.

## GOOD FOR YOU, GOOD FOR THE PLANET

Foraging doesn't even have to take place in the wild, it can start in your own back garden. Let's take the humble dandelion. This widespread, often considered invasive, plant is incredibly important for biodiversity, especially with the loss of wildflower meadows and other sources of food and habitats. Ubiquitous and resilient, dandelions can thrive in the scrappiest lawns and grassland, and take deep root in the poorest soils, and even in the cracks in your patio slabs. If you've ever tried to dig up a dandelion from your garden, roots and all, you'll know just how tenacious they are.

We may disregard dandelions as weeds, but they play a vital role in our ecosystem. Pollinators from bees to beetles love them, while birds enjoy the seeds. They first bloom in early spring before most other flowers are out, making them a vital first food in spring – and a source of joy for children who love to puff away the gossamer seed clocks.

# A SiMPLE SPRiNG SALAD

Combine dandelion leaves with sweeter ingredients in salads to get used to the flavour. Toss with leaves such as butterhead or gem lettuce, a handful of fresh herbs such as mint and oregano, halved cherry tomatoes, toasted pine nuts (or any nuts or seeds you like) and add a drizzle of extra virgin olive oil and balsamic or fruit vinegar.

Dandelions support many ecosystems, and recent research by scientists from five UK universities to assess the benefits of all types of urban land use for pollinators, showed that residential gardens, community gardens and allotments in towns and cities are particularly important for supporting pollinators, revealing that dandelions are one of the key species that support them along with other "weeds" such as brambles, thistles and buttercups, and the herbs lavender and borage.[4]

While these yellow flowers blooming en masse are a welcome sight for wildlife, many people consider them pernicious intruders and ruthlessly eradicate them from lawns and flowerbeds. This is why simply minimizing lawn mowing, especially in spring, and letting weeds do their thing in a corner of your garden is a brilliant "no-effort" way to support biodiversity. In 1878, the philosopher Ralph Waldo Emerson wrote: "What is a weed? A plant whose virtues have not yet been discovered". The virtues of dandelions are not so much undiscovered as forgotten in recent times, as they've long been used in herbal medicine to treat everything from inflammation to kidney problems and high blood pressure. All parts of dandelions are not only safe to eat, they have many culinary and medicinal uses, and there's an argument that dandelions should be recategorized as a herb rather than a weed, although they have no fragrance.

Young dandelion leaves and their flowers can be used in a variety of ways in the kitchen, including in salads, stir-fries, curries and smoothies. The leaves have a spinach-meets-rocket flavour and can be eaten raw or cooked in pretty much any recipe that calls for leafy veg such as spinach or rocket (arugula). They can be a little bitter, although some people find that those picked in shady areas are sweeter than those in full sun. The flowers can be scattered on salads or other dishes, or used to make dandelion vinegar, and both leaves and flower heads can be used to make a tea. Even the root can be eaten – it's often dried and used as a natural coffee alternative, although for anyone thinking of trying it, don't expect it to taste anything like your usual morning cuppa.

Picking these humble little plants from your own lawn may not feel like "proper" foraging, but starting with dandelions can not only add a nutritious new food to your diet, it may lead to further foraging adventures in the wild, helping you connect more deeply with nature and learn to eat in harmony with the seasons.

# NUTRITIONAL NOTES

From root to flower, dandelions are packed with vitamins, minerals, fibre and antioxidants. The flowers are particularly rich in antioxidant polyphenols, which among other health benefits may help to reduce inflammation. Dandelion root is also a rich source of the prebiotic fibre, inulin, which can boost gut health.

## THE FLEDGLING FORAGER'S CALENDAR

Experienced foragers can find something edible in every season, but for the newcomer the peak times are spring to autumn (fall). Here are a few ideas for wild foods to gather that are easy to identify, and both environmentally sustainable and worth the effort of picking. Some of the fruits mentioned here are not technically "wild" as they may have been originally planted by human hand (including tree fruits such as medlar, mulberries and quince), but fruit trees that were once part of orchards or gardens can be found on common land, so it's worth looking out for them.

- **Spring:** dandelion (leaves then flowers), nettles, wild garlic

- **Late Spring/Early Summer:** dandelion (flowers), dulse (seaweed), elderflowers, fennel (flowers), nettles, wild garlic (late spring), wild strawberries, wood sorrel

- **Summer:** bilberries, blackberries, dulse, elderflowers (flowers in early summer, followed by elderberries in late summer), fennel (flowers then seeds), mulberries (late summer), nettles (regrowth), wood sorrel

- **Autumn (Fall):** blackberries, bilberries, crab apples, damsons, dulse, elderberries, fennel (seeds), figs, hazelnuts, juniper berries, medlar, mulberries, nettles (regrowth), plums, quince, rosehips (dog and field roses), sloes (blackthorn), sweet chestnuts, walnuts, wood sorrel

# FORAGING CHALLENGE – 5 TO FIND

When you are ready to move on from nettles and dandelions, here are my five favourite wild ingredients that are easy to identify and have interesting flavours.

## 1 WILD GARLIC (ALLIUM URSINUM)

**In Season:** Spring to early summer.

**How to Find It:** Mostly found in woodlands and shady banks, wild garlic (also known as ramsons) has wide, spear-shaped, soft leaves and white flowers. Easily recognized by the smell – if you're picking wild garlic make sure it has a distinctive garlicky aroma, as to less experienced foragers it can look similar to poisonous Lily of the Valley, which does not smell of garlic.

**Tasting Notes:** Younger leaves and seed pods have a deliciously mild, fresh garlic flavour, but by early summer the taste and texture of the larger leaves starts to become stronger and less pleasant. One of the most versatile of wild ingredients, wild garlic can be used in risotto, pesto, soup and all kinds of dishes. The flowers add beauty and fresh flavour to salads too.

## 2 PINEAPPLEWEED (MATRICARIA DISCOIDEA)

**In Season:** From late spring to autumn (fall).

**How to Find It:** With fuzzy yellow flowers that look a bit like a miniature upside-down pineapple, this small plant is often found in urban landscapes, growing on pathways, roadsides and waste ground. You've probably walked over it many times – and it does taste like pineapple! Roll the flower head between your fingers – if it smells pineapple-y you've identified it correctly, so give it a try.

**Tasting Notes:** You can use the flower heads in a salad – or to make a cordial, jelly or granita.

## 3 WOOD SORREL (OXALIS ACETOSELLA)

**In Season:** Late spring to mid-summer is peak picking time, when the young leaves are most succulent.

**How to Find It:** Spotting a carpet of wood sorrel is often a sign you are walking in ancient woodland and it's distinguishable from clover by its heart-shaped leaves and red stems.

**Tasting Notes:** This tangy, almost lemony-tasting leaf contains oxalates that are not good for the liver in vast quantities, but a scattering of the leaves and flowers on a salad is delicious.

## 4 ELDERFLOWERS (SAMBUCUS NIGRA)

**In Season:** Late spring to mid-summer.

**How to Find It:** These creamy white flowers can be spotted along roadsides, in parks, waste ground and along canals. Easy to identify by their saucer-sized clusters of flowers and distinctive scent, these are so easy to pick, but avoid any with brown flowers or that are covered in black fly.

**Tasting Notes:** The flower heads make excellent dessert fritters, or use to make a simple cordial that can be added to everything from cocktails to cakes. Look out for the berries later in the summer, which are also delicious in a spiced syrup for drizzling on desserts, for fruit vinegar or even a homemade wine.

## 5 BLACKTHORN (PRUNUS SPINOSA)

**In Season:** Sloe berries can be picked throughout autumn (fall).

**How to Find It:** Look in hedgerows, wasteland and along footpaths, canals and old railway lines. The berries look like little round plums and the branches are almost black in colour. Watch out for the rather lethal thorns.

**Tasting Notes:** Sloes taste pretty astringent when raw and are mainly gathered for one reason only – for making sloe gin, although you can make a lovely jam with them too. For gin, mix together 500g (1lb 2oz) washed and de-stemmed sloes, 250g (9oz) caster (superfine) sugar and 1 litre (34fl oz) gin and pour into 2 clean jars. Seal and leave to marinade in a dark place for at least 3 months (afficionados recommend a minimum of 6 months), then strain through muslin, rebottle and leave to mature again for as long as you have the patience, for a deeply flavourful fruity tipple.

# A NOTE ON SAFETY

While you can safely eat dandelions and daisies, buttercups should never be eaten – despite their associations with butter – as they contain ranunculin, which when crushed or chewed becomes the toxin protoanemonin. This may cause blistering inside your mouth and severe digestive irritation. They are particularly toxic for horses, dogs and cats.

The type and availability of wild foods you can pick is dependent on the season, and also on the country in which you live. Plant identification apps can be useful, but they are not always accurate, so it's best to have a reliable colour-illustrated field guide in your pocket. Foraging courses are a great way to build confidence in identifying wild foods.

Mushrooms require expertise to identify accurately (which is why I've not listed any in the calendar) and I recommend that you never eat any wild fungi unless you are absolutely certain what type they are. As with all wild foods, if in any doubt, don't eat it, as some plants can be very harmful to health. Extra caution is recommended when eating foraged foods if you have any underlying health conditions or are pregnant.

Finally, remember to only forage in public places or get permission from the landowner to go foraging on private property.

# AN ACQUiRED TASTE

Our hunter-gatherer ancestors didn't have refined sugar and the only sweetness in their diet came from wild berries and a little honey. The bitter or sharp flavours of some wild foods can be surprising and even a little unpleasant at first to those who eat a lot of sweet foods (which these days is most of us). These flavours are part of a clever defence mechanism developed by many plants to deter creatures from eating them, although the tactic has backfired in some respects as the compounds that produce these bitter flavours, and which are often toxic to insects, often make them more nutritious to humans, such as glucosinolates in broccoli, sprouts and kale. Many wild foods might be regarded as an "acquired taste" and we must train our tastebuds to appreciate them. After all, polyphenol-rich, naturally bitter foods such as red wine, coffee and dark chocolate are surprisingly easy for humans to become accustomed to.

# SIGNPOSTS

For more on:

🌱 **Gut health,** *see* **chapters 3 and 7**

🌱 **Herbs,** *see* **chapter 4**

🌱 **Further reading on foraging,** *see* **chapters 1 and 6**

# FORAGER'S MUFFINS

*Great for serving with soup, these vegan savoury muffins are a lovely way to cook with nettles. They also work with baby spinach leaves and you could add some dandelion leaves too. Best served warm.*

**Makes 6 | Prep time: 15 minutes | Cooking time: 20 minutes**

## INGREDIENTS

20g (¾oz) chia seeds

80ml (2¾fl oz) water

1 tablespoon olive oil

40g (1½oz) red onion, finely diced

1 garlic clove, minced

50g (2oz) nettle leaves, washed and finely sliced

125g (4oz) plain (all-purpose) flour

2 level teaspoons baking powder

sea salt and freshly ground black pepper

50g (2oz) sundried tomatoes, drained and finely chopped

1 tablespoon balsamic vinegar

80ml (2¾fl oz) plant-based milk (soya or almond)

## METHOD

Preheat the oven to 200°C (400°F/gas mark 6). Line a 6-hole muffin tin with paper cases.

Place the chia seeds and water in a bowl and set aside to soak.

Heat the olive oil in a large pan over a low heat, add the red onion and garlic and gently sauté for 5–7 minutes until the onion is soft and translucent but not burned. Add the nettle leaves and continue to sauté until thoroughly wilted, then remove from the heat.

Put the flour and baking powder in a bowl, season with a pinch of salt and some black pepper and mix well.

Drain the chia seed mixture and add to a separate bowl, then add the sundried tomatoes, balsamic vinegar, nettle mixture and plant milk and mix until well combined. Add to the dry ingredients and combine thoroughly.

Divide the mixture between the muffin cases. Bake in the oven for 20 minutes until beautifully risen and golden brown. Serve warm.

# 13

# SELF-CARE INSPIRED BY NATURE

"Consumers have not been told effectively enough that they have huge power and that purchasing and shopping involve a moral choice."

Anita Roddick, founder of *The Body Shop*

**THE GOAL:**
**TO CREATE A NURTURING PLANT-CENTRED BEAUTY RITUAL**

**B**EAUTY ISN'T SKIN-DEEP – IT COMES FROM WITHIN, NOT FROM magic potions and lotions created in a lab. Staying hydrated and eating a nutritious, plant-rich diet is absolutely the best way to get glowing skin, shiny hair and strong nails. When you start living plantfully and eating a predominantly wholefood plant-based diet, you'll soon realize there's a close link between ingredients you use in the kitchen, or even pick from the garden and out in the wild, and the ingredients that nourish your skin, hair and nails too. If you're naturally eating a skin-sustaining diet packed with fibre, antioxidant polyphenols, vitamins, minerals and essential fatty acids, these are all the ingredients you need to maintain a healthy gut and get a gorgeous glow from the inside out. Even if you have a skin condition or tend to get breakouts, taking a look at diet and lifestyle factors can really make a difference to skin health, especially in combination with your prescribed treatments. A healthy diet, regular exercise and staying hydrated are the foundation of any beauty regime – more important than any beauty products – perhaps with the exception of sunscreen.

Skincare therapist, natural beauty expert and author Jess Arnaudin agrees. "Your skin is your body's largest organ and it reflects your inner health and what's going on internally. You can be using the best organic plant-based skincare, but if you're loading up on highly processed, sugary junk all day then your skin won't be glowing with health. Oxidation happens throughout our body and on our skin, and it can affect the skin's barrier if you are not getting enough antioxidants, which means minor breakout healing can really slow down. So, fill up your plate with lots of fresh, vibrant, minimally processed foods, so your whole body, including your skin, can function optimally."

Throughout this book I've been encouraging you to live and shop more mindfully, to embrace the healing powers of nature and to build a healthy diet from the ground up. The same is true for your beauty regime. When you break down the barrier between products you use in the bathroom and those you cook with in the kitchen, you'll discover that many plant foods are not only beneficial when ingested, but also when applied directly to the skin. Berries, fruit, vegetables, juices and plant oils all contain ingredients that help promote healthy skin and hair when applied topically. And what could be more fun than popping on a quick anti-inflammatory homemade strawberry face mask while you enjoy a smoothie in the garden? Simply mash 3–4 strawberries with a little coconut yoghurt and a drizzle of honey, then apply. This is just one of many beautifully simple ideas to try that connect nutritious food with a nourishing beauty regime.

# FOODiE BEAUTY TRiCKS

Jess Arnaudin suggests some of her favourite quick fixes to try next time you're in the kitchen:

- If you're cooking with olive, coconut or avocado oil, rub a little into your hands or cuticles to give them some love while you work.

- When making avocado on toast, use the other half of the avocado to make a very simple face mask with some coconut yoghurt.

- If there's a little bit of smoothie left in the blender, mix it with some rice bran or oat powder and make it into a paste, then scrub it onto your skin for a natural exfoliator.

- Grapes are naturally rich in alpha hydroxy acids, so give yourself a little lip treatment: slice a grape in half and rub the cut side onto your lips to enjoy the skin softening benefits on chapped lips.

## UGLY ON THE INSIDE

The big brands have cottoned on to the fact that we like the idea of using more natural, plant-based ingredients, and will often mention that their products contain "superfoods" such as avocado or quinoa, or use vague terms such as "botanicals" on their labelling. But the amount of those ingredients in each product is often miniscule. Yet, here's the thing – even though many of us love the idea of being more natural with our grooming, deep down many of us have trust issues with natural plant-based beauty products, fearing they won't be as effective as our tried-and-tested brands, perhaps because we feel they don't have the benefits of the latest science or technology, or we feel anxious about changing a beauty routine we've been comfortable with for many years.

It might help to remember that many commercial and more natural brands often use the same active plant ingredients such as fruit enzymes, vitamins A, C and E, polyphenols, carotenoids, and alpha hydroxy acids (AHAs) because they are extremely effective. These are still chemicals, of course, but they are nourishing, natural, plant-derived chemicals that have been proven to be safe and effective over many years. Any trust issues should be with the multinational cosmetic companies who sell bottles of goop that over-promise and under-deliver, and which contain a whole load of other things we don't need to absorb into our bodies.

What you won't find in good quality natural brands is the extra fillers, synthetic fragrances, preservatives, emulsifiers and additives that are there purely to extend the shelf life and improve the texture and consistency of the product. Without all these, many natural products are often more concentrated and more powerful. Yes, some can be more expensive, but thanks to the provenance and potency of the ingredients, a little tends to go a long way – and the price per use is reduced.

In some cases, you do have to make an adjustment to your expectations because without all those added extras, natural products may have a different texture or may need to be used in a different way to what you are used to, but with so much innovation in this market, it's possible to find products that feel luxurious, smell incredible and perform brilliantly too.

Think about it like this: buying traditional commercial products and applying them to your body is the beauty equivalent of buying a readymade meal or TV dinner. There may be some benefits at a basic level – the meal will satisfy your hunger, the shampoo will clean your hair – but the negatives such as the unnecessary and unhealthy ingredients in that product, not to mention the single-use plastic packaging, almost certainly outweigh them.

When you start shopping more mindfully for food, you'll find you also start thinking differently about other buying decisions and it's inevitable that you might start to feel it doesn't make sense to buy an organic veg box to avoid consuming pesticides and be kinder to the planet, while still buying beauty products that contain carcinogenic and hormone-disrupting chemicals, or ingredients that fuel climate change such as unsustainably-sourced palm oil or petrochemicals.

The global beauty industry is huge – it's expected to generate over £615 billion (US$824 billion) by 2025,[1] which means it's incredibly important that we show our preference for more sustainable, organic, plant-based products by supporting brands that produce them. Social media has allowed many of these new independent brands to flourish without the huge ad spend of the big corporates, and the organic and natural beauty sector is growing faster than ever.[2]

It's a trend not only driven by the desire to live less wastefully and combat climate change, but also growing concerns about just how many chemicals we're exposed to daily. You may think that ingesting chemicals from food is potentially more harmful than using moisturizer or shower gel, but it's been estimated that every morning, the average woman will apply 12 different products to her skin and hair, which equates to at least 126 different chemicals. All that before you've even had your morning cup of coffee.

When you combine this with chemicals from the hundreds of other food-based, household and environmental pollutants we are exposed to every day, it's no wonder this "human toxome" is increasingly being linked by scientists to a range of serious diseases. Even where chemicals have been deemed safe by regulatory bodies and are used at permitted levels in products, we don't yet fully understand the impact of this layering of multiple chemicals and their accumulation in us and in ecosystems over time. While using one product containing an infinitesimally small amount of a paraben is not necessarily going to be a big issue, when we are using these ingredients across multiple products for a whole lifetime, it creates a significant toxic load in our bodies.

It's extraordinary that products designed to make us look more beautiful on the outside can be so ugly on the inside. "I think we will look back and shudder at what we used to put on our bodies," says Jess Arnaudin. "Our skin is a beautiful barrier protecting us from the outside world, but it's absorbent. It's the reason you can use a nicotine or birth control patch: your skin drinks it up and something systemically will change within you because of the chemicals in that patch. It's the same with the beauty products we apply to our skin."

Even knowing all this about conventional beauty products, many of us can still be very reluctant to part with our old favourites – or to give up the thrill of discovering new ones. Add on the enticement of celebrity endorsement and all the beauty influencers recommending the latest "it" product, and soon these beautifully packed bottles of promises are flying off the shelves and into our makeup bags – until the next big thing is launched. Products manufactured and marketed by the big brands are so popular not necessarily because they are any more effective, but because they are big spenders on promotion. In 2020, cosmetic and perfume companies spent £2.8 billion (US$3.7 billion) on advertising in the USA alone.[3] With this level of bombardment, it's hard not to be seduced.

# DECODING THE LABELS

The answer, of course, is to start thinking plantfully: buying products made from sustainably sourced, renewable and organic plant ingredients – which are going to be much better from a health, ethical and planetary perspective – and combining them with a few homemade remedies too. Look for products that use plant oils such as shea butter, which are fragranced with pure essential oils and use simple kitchen or innovative recycled waste ingredients, such as sugar or coffee grounds. Simple switches, such as making your own face masks from kitchen ingredients or choosing products with a simpler ingredients list, like natural face, body or hair oils rather than moisturizers or leave-in conditioner, can quickly make your bathroom cabinet look a lot more plantful.

Cosmetic marketing and product labelling can be pretty sneaky, so you always need to read labels with a cynical eye. When we talk about ethical beauty, conversations around issues such as animal welfare, harmful chemicals and sustainability can become intermingled, and it's not always easy to find products that tick all the boxes. For example, an organic lip balm may contain animal ingredients, while a purely plant-based product may include some ingredients from an unethical supply chain or that have been farmed unsustainably. Whether it's more important to you that your products are vegan, organic, ethical or eco-friendly comes down to your own values hierarchy, but the holy grail is to find brands that are kind to animals, people and planet.

As there are currently no legal definitions for how terms such as "natural", "green", "eco" or "clean" can be used on beauty packaging, products with these words on the label may still contain synthetic dyes, preservatives or fragrances, petrochemicals, harmful chemicals or ingredients tested on animals, so always check the ingredients list on the back of the pack before being charmed by the promises on the front.

## ORGANIC

A certified organic beauty product means that it uses no GM ingredients, no controversial chemicals, no parabens or phthalates, no synthetic colours, dyes or fragrances, no nanoparticles, certified sustainable palm oil, no animal testing, and recycled and recyclable packaging wherever possible. Depending on where you live, choosing certified organic products – such as those with the USDA certified organic seal, the Soil Association symbol in the UK and the international COSMOS symbol – means that at least 95% of the ingredients of that product must be organic.

However, unlike with food products, "organic" is not a protected term on cosmetics so anyone can put it on a label. Some small independent brands may not have the budget to go through the certification process, but are genuinely organic, so it's worth doing some research.

## NATURAL/GREEN/SUSTAINABLE/CLEAN/WILD-CRAFTED/BOTANICAL/FORAGED/HOLISTIC

I've lumped all these together because there's no regulation for the use of any of these terms on beauty and wellbeing products, and while some may be genuine descriptions of a product's contents, in other cases it could be "greenwashing". An uncertified product could have just 1% natural ingredients and would be able to use the word "natural" on the label. You must also consider how the product is made – for example, poorly processed natural ingredients such as plant oils or plant extracts will be less effective if subjected to high heat, while "wild-crafted" or "foraged" ingredients irresponsibly harvested may damage ecosystems. In the US, the FDA has not defined the meaning of "natural" and so can't regulate the validity of these claims on labels. Keep your "marketing hocus pocus" radar on high alert and choose brands that are really transparent about their sourcing.

## VEGAN OR CRUELTY-FREE?

These terms are often used interchangeably but they are not the same thing. A product labelled as "cruelty-free" (look for the internationally recognized leaping bunny logo for certified products) means neither the final product nor any of the ingredients have been tested on animals and includes products that are not sold in countries where post-market animal testing is required by law, such as China, which is a big ethical issue for products made by some leading global brands. However, cruelty-free products could still contain animal ingredients such as honey or milk. Products labelled – and ideally independently certified – as vegan contain no animal-derived ingredients and are also cruelty-free.

## FAIRWILD CERTIFICATION

The global certification from the FairWild Foundation is a good one to look out for, as it guarantees best practice in land management in the harvesting of wild plant ingredients, and ensures fair treatment, working conditions and pay for workers.

# 3 QUICK KITCHEN BEAUTY TREATS

### 1 Soothing Eye Mask

For tired, puffy, irritated eyes, brew yourself a pot of antioxidant-rich green tea using two teabags. Leave the bags to cool while you enjoy your tea, then pop the bags on your eyes for 10 minutes while you take a time-out. The caffeine in the tea can reduce puffiness, while the antioxidant flavonoids and tannins can tighten the skin and draw out fluid. It's thought green tea (and rooibos works too, if you prefer a caffeine-free brew) can reduce the appearance of wrinkles.

### 2 Herby Salt Scrub

Sea salt is a fantastic natural body exfoliator (although generally too abrasive for the face). Mix 120g (4oz) finely ground sea salt with 3 teaspoons oil (try olive, jojoba, avocado or almond) and 15–20 drops of essential oils (try a combination of favourites such as eucalyptus, mint, lemon, orange, sage, lavender), and a few fresh herbs for extra zing, such as mint, lavender or sage. Add a little more oil if the texture is too dry. Pop the mixture in a sterilized jar and it will keep for a couple of months. Hop in a nice steamy shower and when your skin is warm and your pores are opened, apply to your skin in a gentle circular motion. Rinse off thoroughly.

### 3 Refreshing Foot Soak

Add around 120g (4oz) bicarbonate of soda (baking soda) to a washing-up bowl of warm water and stir until dissolved. Add 2–3 drops of peppermint essential oil and soak your feet for around 30 minutes. Rinse and pat dry your feet, then apply a plant-based foot moisturizer.

# THE 5-STEP DETOX

If you're looking to live more plantfully when it comes to your self-care routine, think of it as a positive opportunity to break out of a beauty rut. When you shake things up and switch to plant-based products, your skin, hair and nails will thank you for it.

Jess Arnaudin recommends creating a mindful, relaxing beauty ritual that you can really look forward to each morning and evening. "This is an opportunity to transform a change that may feel overwhelming at first into a really beautiful moment of sensory joy," says Jess. "There's no way I can go to sleep without doing my skincare ritual, it's such a sacred bookend to my day. If you're not looking forward to using your products each day, you're using the wrong things."

Living more sustainably generally means getting used to buying less "stuff" and this applies to self-care too. Consider if you really need so many beauty products in the first place. We're often fed ideas such as a "12-step beauty regime", for example, but this is a marketing strategy to make us buy more products. Start by replacing your most-used and essential daily products as they run out with plant-based, sustainable alternatives, and look for versatile, multi-purpose products that have two or three uses, such as a beauty balm. Some products might not need to be replaced at all. Aim to support brands that are plant-based, sustainable and ethical all along the chain, from ingredient sourcing to product development to manufacturing, packaging and distribution.

To get you started, here's a five-step process to going natural. I know, that does sound like a conventional beauty marketing message, doesn't it? But this is not a hollow promise, it really will change your skin and health for the better.

## 1 NEVER SKIMP ON SUNSCREEN

If you're not already using this daily all year round, make this the first thing you change, as not only does it keep you safe from dangerous UV exposure, but sun damage also causes premature ageing. From an eco-perspective, 14,000 tonnes of sunscreen ends up in the sea every year, where it can harm microorganisms and damage coral.[4] Some studies suggest there's no such thing as perfectly reef-safe sunscreen, but you should certainly avoid anything containing oxybenzone, octinoxate, octocrylene, petrochemicals, parabens or propylene glycol, and look for a vegan-friendly mineral formulation with zinc and titanium oxides, plus antioxidants to provide extra protection for your skin.

It's worth mentioning nanoparticles here, as some sunscreens (and other cosmetic and food products) use these extremely small particles – in the case of sunscreen it's zinc and titanium oxides – in their formulations. There is some concern that the small size of nanoparticles makes it possible for us (and wildlife) to inhale or ingest them, or for them to pass through the blood stream into our cells, where they may create chemical reactions that have molecular and genetic effects that could be harmful, especially in combination with other toxic substances. As we don't yet fully understand the potential long-term risks of nanoparticles, they are best avoided.

## 2 AVOID SYNTHETIC FRAGRANCE

Synthetic fragrances can contain anything up to 200 ingredients, which don't have to be disclosed on the label as fragrance formulas are considered to be "trade secrets". Some of these compounds are known to be a cause of indoor air pollution and are associated with a wide range of health risks from immune-system damage to hormone disruption, neurotoxicity (damaging for the brain), and increasing the growth of oestrogen-responsive breast cancer cells, as well as being toxic for aquatic life in waterways and oceans.

Often found in synthetic fragrances, phthalates have been known to be a problematic ingredient for a long time. Many are endocrine-disrupting chemicals that have been linked with issues such as reproductive defects, infertility and cancer. While many are now banned, some are still out there in everyday products, so always choose fragrance-free products, avoid anything with "Fragrance" or "Parfum" on the ingredients list and steer clear of anything containing dibutyl, diethylhexyl and diethyl phthalates. When you switch, artificial scents soon seem cheap and overpowering compared to products harnessing the natural aromas of plant essential oils.

# PLASTIC WATCH

Did you know that on average, every one of us absorbs up to 5g of plastic every week?[5] That's around the amount used to make a credit card. This is largely from the tonnes of solid microplastic particles and liquid polymers found in cosmetics. It's thought that every second skin and haircare product contains at least one plastic polymer that is known to be harmful to the environment, and these build up in our bodies, soil and water, remaining in our ecosystems for many years with unknown consequences.

## 3 SWITCH DEODORANT

This can be one of the hardest swaps, but is one of the most important. Many deodorants contain parabens as preservatives, while aluminium-based ingredients in conventional antiperspirants prevent sweating by clogging pores, which some experts believe may be harmful for our health. Natural deodorants do work differently and you may have to get used to feeling some moisture under your arms, but they use plant compounds to combat sweat smells along with naturally absorbent ingredients such as baking soda and arrowroot. It can take trial and error to find a brand that works for you, but it's well worth the effort.

## 4 BE KINDER TO YOUR SKIN

Skin is our biggest organ, and if you're looking to detoxify your regime, focus first on anything that is applied to your skin, especially if it's left to soak in. You'll want to start avoiding mineral oil or other petroleum-derived ingredients along with skin-stripping SLS (sodium lauryl sulphate) and SLES (sodium laureth sulphate), which can be found in anything that foams or bubbles. These cheap surfactants (which means they provide a foaming or emulsifying effect) weaken your skin's natural protective barrier. A product doesn't need to foam to be effective, we've just been conditioned to equate bubbles with cleanliness.

Parabens are well publicized as beauty product villains and thankfully many products are now being marketed as "paraben-free". These preservatives are still absolutely everywhere though, despite scientific studies suggesting these oestrogen-mimicking chemicals can disrupt hormones in the body, affect fertility and increase the risk of cancer, particularly breast cancer. Avoid anything with the -paraben suffix on the ingredients list such as methylparaben or isobutylparaben.

## 5 FIND A TRUSTED OUTLET

It's a good idea to find an online store that specializes in vegan, natural, sustainable and organic products as a starting point – at least you know everything they stock will already tick many of the boxes for being eco, cruelty-free, plant-based and non-toxic. Look for sample sizes or gift sets to try different products before committing to full sizes.

---

## SWEET DREAMS BATH SALTS

*Jess Arnaudin has kindly shared her favourite sleep-boosting bath soak, which makes enough for two baths. It's safe for children too.*

---

**YOU WILL NEED**

1 cup Epsom salts

1 cup baking soda

½ cup carrier oil (grapeseed is nice and light, but you can use any oil such as avocado, sweet almond or olive)

8 drops of mandarin essential oil

4 drops of lavender essential oil

4 drops of sandalwood essential oil

**METHOD**

1 Mix all the ingredients thoroughly and keep in a jar until ready to use.

**HOW TO USE**

Pour half the jar of salts into warm running water, then relax in the bath for at least 20 minutes to get the full benefits of trans-dermal magnesium absorption from the salts.
Have sweet dreams.

## ROSE AND YLANG YLANG FACE MIST

*Rosewater is gentle, hydrating and calms redness. It has antibacterial effects and, in combination with antioxidant-rich vitamin E oil, helps protect your skin from environmental damage. I find a spritz of this uplifts my mood too.*

**For a 100ml (3½fl oz) glass spray bottle**

**YOU WILL NEED**

a few drops of pure organic vitamin E oil

3 drops of ylang ylang organic essential oil

50ml (1¾fl oz) organic rose water

**METHOD**

1 Simply combine all the ingredients in a glass spray bottle, give it a little shake to mix and you are ready to spray.

**HOW TO USE**

You can use your mist to hydrate your skin and hair during the day, to freshen your makeup or to mist your face after cleansing before applying a plant-based facial oil. Your skin benefits from lots of lovely hydration and nutrients when the water and oil are applied together.

## SIGNPOSTS

For more on:

🌱 **Easy ways to eat more plants, see chapter 7**

🌱 **Harmful chemicals in the home, see chapter 14**

# 14

# HOW GREEN IS YOUR CLEAN?

"The objective of cleaning is not just to clean, but to feel happiness living within that environment."

Marie Kondo

**THE GOAL:**
**TO MAKE YOUR FIRST HOMEMADE CLEANING PRODUCT**

**I**F YOU'RE THE SORT OF PERSON WHO PREFERS TO MAKE YOUR own pasta sauce because it's more economical, uses fresh, natural ingredients and is better for your health – or at least, if you aspire to be that person – then for the exact same reasons you should consider making your own cleaning products. Every time you spray something in your home, the chemicals it contains will end up in your body either by ingesting, inhaling or absorption through the skin. These toxins pollute the atmosphere and when they are washed down the drain, end up in waterways and eventually the sea. For example, when sodium hypochlorite, the active ingredient in bleach, mixes in water with other chemicals it produces chlorine compounds such as dioxins, which are not only harmful to marine life and other wildlife but also for humans, and they remain in the environment for a very long time. Modern cleaning is a surprisingly dirty business.

By contrast, natural cleaning is clean in every sense of the word, using gentler chemicals and kitchen ingredients to achieve the same sparkling finish, but without polluting your home or the environment. As with beauty products, there can be an element of mistrust when it comes to natural cleaning – people worry that products such as vinegar or bicarbonate of soda can't truly achieve the same level of cleanliness, especially in a world that has become a little too obsessed with eliminating germs with antibacterial products. But natural cleaning recipes are not only just as effective in most cases as commercial products, but they are also actually fun to make – it's a little like conducting your own science experiments, trying out different combinations to see which formulas work best for you. If you're growing your own herbs, it's lovely to be able use some of these in your cleaning recipes, while kitchen scraps such as citrus fruit peels have so many uses too.

# GET READY FOR A FRESH, GREEN CLEAN

It's time to think more plantfully about cleaning. The best way to get your floors clean enough to eat your dinner from is to use everyday ingredients – some of which you could safely eat – although you wouldn't necessarily want to. If you're ready to start adding some homemade products to your cleaning repertoire, the simplest way to make a transition is when you notice a particular product is running out, to make a plan to replace it with something more natural. It might feel like you're adding to your already busy workload by having to find time to make cleaning potions on top of everything else you're juggling, but many of the most effective recipes are so simple, once you have a few basic ingredients in stock, they take only a minute to put together and one product can often have several uses – for example citric acid can be used for descaling a kettle and cleaning a toilet.

For almost every job around the home, there's an effective homemade recipe that will work just as well as a commercial product. Wendy Graham, author and green lifestyle blogger at moralfibres.co.uk, says she's only found a couple of exceptions. After many years of experimenting with a variety of concoctions, the perfect dishwashing product has so far eluded her – although there's nothing to stop you trying to come up with your own recipes. "I have tried and failed to make an effective washing-up liquid and an effective dishwasher detergent," she says. "My efforts literally and figuratively don't cut the mustard. I have done some research and found that the ingredients required to achieve good dishwashing results are heavily restricted. So, I say when it comes to dishwashing, save yourself the hassle and buy readymade eco-friendly options instead."

# YOUR GREEN CLEANING PANTRY

As you gradually get through all your bottles of commercial sprays and liquids, you can start building your pantry of non-toxic cleaning ingredients, many of which are very versatile and can be used in a variety of different ways. If you bulk buy the ingredients online, you can not only save money, but also reduce the amount of plastic packaging that gets thrown away, as you can recycle and reuse old spray bottles for your own mixtures.

When you buy your essential ingredients in bulk, decanting them into beautiful bottles and jars (ideally recycled ones) and making attractive labels can really make your cleaning supplies look stylish enough to keep on display – unlike most shop-bought products with their plastic containers and gaudy branding.

The ingredients you will need depend on the recipes you decide to use, but these are some of the most useful things to keep in stock:

- **White Vinegar**: A multipurpose, non-toxic base for many different cleaning recipes.

- **Coarse Salt**: A brilliant natural scourer, salt is great for scrubbing pans and chopping boards.

- **Bicarbonate of Soda (Baking Soda)**: Another staple in many recipes, and often much cheaper bought in bulk from hardware shops or online.

- **Liquid Castile Soap**: Made from plant oils, this simple, biodegradable soap is very versatile. It's more expensive than some staples on this list, but it can be bought in large bottles and used diluted to make it stretch.

- **Glycerine**: Made from plant oils, glycerine is a natural thickener (you've probably used it in baking or for icing/frosting) and it's handy for emulsifying essential oils with water for homemade cleaning sprays and air fresheners.

- **Borax Substitute**: A cheap ingredient that's useful for general cleaning and laundry, especially tougher cleaning jobs like tiles and toilets.

- **Hydrogen Peroxide**: A very effective disinfectant and a safer, more eco-friendly alternative to bleach, which kills germs by oxidation.

- **Citric Acid**: Great for tackling limescale in kitchens and bathrooms, this highly concentrated fruit acid can be very potent and needs careful handling. Even natural cleaning ingredients can be dangerous if not used properly.

- **Soda Crystals (Washing Soda)**: A cheap and cheerful multipurpose cleaner, soda crystals are versatile for general cleaning and laundry.

- **Vodka**: Great for degreasing and deodorizing, just buy the cheapest supermarket own-brand bottle you can find. Save the good stuff for cocktails.

- **Pure Essential Oils**: These can be expensive but are a good investment if you like cleaning products with a lovely fragrance. You only need 2–3 oils – lavender, tea tree and either lemon or sweet orange would be a good basic collection to start you off. Alternatively, you can use fresh herbs and citrus fruits to add a delicious aroma to your products.

- **Kitchen Staples**: Olive oil, lemons, oranges and fresh herbs are all useful.

## A NOTE ON SAFETY

Remember that many natural cleaning ingredients are still chemicals and can be dangerous if used incorrectly. Always research recipes from reliable sources and check before mixing ingredients, as the mixture may be either harmful or ineffective. For example, mixing hydrogen peroxide and vinegar produces peracetic acid, which is damaging to lungs and can trigger allergies.

Also, some ingredients such as citrus oils and vinegar may damage natural materials such as stone, granite and marble tiles or worktops.

If there's one stalwart of the green cleaning repertoire, it's white vinegar. Wendy Graham admits that vinegar can be a stumbling block for some people when they first try natural cleaning. "Vinegar is an excellent and cheap natural cleaning product, but the downside is that it does smell of, well, vinegar," she says. "The good news is that there are ways around this. I mostly use vinegar diluted in water in a 50/50 ratio, so it's not so strong.

You can also add your favourite essential oils to vinegar, or my favourite thrifty method is to infuse vinegar with herbs from the garden and fruit peelings such as orange or lemon rind. It's also important to remember that vinegar is odourless when dry, so the smell never lingers." If you're really not keen on vinegar, there are lots of different natural cleaning products and methods you can use that are vinegar-free, which will still give you great results.

Perhaps Wendy's best tip is to not fall into the common trap of mixing vinegar with bicarbonate of soda (baking soda). "Incorrect recipes may result in ineffective products," she says. "Many cleaning blogs recommend mixing vinegar and bicarbonate of soda (baking soda) together, which despite all the bubbling and fizzing only results in a weak saltwater solution, which won't clean anything well."

While it can be a little acrid when you first spray it, eau de vinegar is at least harmless, unlike the smell of some commercial cleaning products. Fragrances are among the big selling points of commercial brands, marketed as "lemon-fresh" or "coconut bliss". We've become accustomed to associating cleanliness with the aromas of scented bleach, the potent disinfectant smell of anti-bac sprays or the exotic floral fragrance of fabric softener on our bed linen. But most of these aromas are completely synthetic and may signal the presence of potentially toxic chemicals – there's nothing remotely fresh about that "meadow" scent. Our sense of smell is activated by the presence of microscopic particles of a substance in our nose, which means by the time you can smell something, you've already breathed it in. As Chris Woodford says in his book, *Breathless – why air pollution matters and how it affects you*, "If you can smell it, and it's been made in a factory, there's a good chance it's pollution."[1]

This is why it's so important to retrain ourselves to appreciate the natural aroma of our homes without commercial cleaning products, synthetic fragrances or petroleum-based scented candles, knowing we are being kinder to our health if we use safe products such as pure essential oils, fresh lemons or bicarbonate of soda (baking soda) to keep things smelling fresh.

# QUICK WAYS TO USE VINEGAR AND BICARBONATE OF SODA

Even without the complete pantry of natural cleaning products, there's so much you can do with just white vinegar and bicarbonate of soda (baking soda).

## VINEGAR

**Fabric Softener:** Your fabric softener may not be vegan or vegetarian, thanks to the common use of tallow, an animal fat. Using fabric softener also adds unnecessary chemicals to your clothes, towels and bed linens and makes them less absorbent, so over time they can't be washed effectively. It also clogs up your machine and leads to bacterial growth and more bad smells. White vinegar is an ideal alternative, just use the same quantity as you would conventional softener, and add a couple of drops of pure essential oil if you prefer a fragrance. Even without adding any oil, there's no vinegary after-aroma.

**Shower Screen Cleaner:** Undiluted vinegar is great for cleaning soap and limescale from glass shower screens. Spray on, leave for a few minutes and rinse off with warm water and a cotton rag.

**Sponge Sanitizing:** Kill bugs in cloths and sponges by soaking in full-strength vinegar for 5 minutes, then rinse.

## BICARBONATE OF SODA (BAKING SODA)

**Fabric Freshener:** To naturally deodorize carpets, upholstery and mattresses, sprinkle the dry fabric with bicarbonate of soda and leave to absorb, ideally overnight or for as long as possible. Then, hoover thoroughly. You can also mix essential oils into the bicarbonate of soda to leave a lovely fragrance behind.

**Fridge Deodorizer:** Keep your fridge smelling sweet by keeping a small open bowl of bicarbonate of soda at the back, changing it every 3 months.

**Stain Remover:** Make a paste of bicarbonate of soda and water and apply to red wine stains. Leave for a few hours, rinse and wash. This mixture may also work for greasy stains.

# THE TRUE COST OF CLEANING

The idea of saving money is perhaps the biggest personal incentive for going natural. Conventional cleaning is an expensive business, and if you look under your kitchen sink, you'll probably find at least 10–20 different products in there, from laundry liquid to stain removers and glass cleaner. How much do you think you spend on all those chemical concoctions every year, many of which are rarely used? The global household cleaning product industry is expected to be worth £239 billion (US$320 billion) by 2028,[2] so it's understandable that the big brands don't want us to catch onto the fact that relatively cheap ingredients such as vinegar and bicarbonate of soda (baking soda) can do the job just as well, with fewer harmful side effects.

Most people, when they start thinking about switching to greener cleaning, tend to look for commercially produced eco or organic brands first, which is a brilliant step in the right direction. But, in a growing market there's a lot of money to be made from ethically minded consumers, and unfortunately some of the most popular "green" cleaning brands are produced by multinationals that have seized on a fantastic business opportunity while not being at all eco-friendly at heart and they may support animal testing and produce other brands of not-so-green cleaning products. If you are buying commercial eco cleaning products, it's worth checking the credentials of the parent company for their track record on sustainability and animal testing, or supporting an independent brand using vegan-friendly and sustainable plant-based formulas.

Cleaning influencers have become incredibly powerful too, sharing their favourite household hacks on social media with their legions of fans, and sales of products they recommend can soar. Rarely do these influencers share tips for natural methods, however, which are surely the best hacks of all. Wendy believes the reason for this is simple: "There's a lot of money to be made for influencers who can tap into the colossal advertising budgets of multinationals with portfolios of cleaning products. With natural methods, there isn't any financial incentive for influencers; there are no lucrative partnership or sponsorship deals to be struck if they promote unbranded natural ingredients."

# HOW CLEAN DO WE REALLY NEED TO BE?

If you've ever bought a cleaning spray, an oven cleaning kit or bleach-based product and been overpowered by the choking, abrasive fumes, that's the smell of pollution caused by volatile organic compounds (VOCs), chemicals that quickly evaporate in the air. VOCs found in cleaning products can include hazardous chemicals with no safe level of exposure. If there are warning messages on the product to "only use in a well-ventilated room" for example, that's a sure sign there's something in the bottle you don't want to expose yourself or your family to. VOCs also chemically react with other pollutants like ozone and fine particulates, making them linger even longer. So, while we're merrily scrubbing away at dirt, dust and bacteria, we're potentially replacing them with substances that may be much more harmful for health. Chemicals that have been linked to a range of serious health issues from hormone disruption to cancer are also regularly found in cleaning products.[3] Sites such as ethicalconsumer.org and ewg.org are great resources for running background checks on both the ethics of brands and potentially harmful ingredients used in products.

The global Covid-19 pandemic has further fuelled the antibacterial trend, but big brands have long played on consumers' fears about the hidden threat of bacteria in our homes, adding antibacterial chemicals not just to surface cleaners but to products such as washing-up and laundry liquids, where they serve no purpose at all because hot water and soap will effectively kill any bugs.

It's important to understand the difference between cleaning and sanitizing. A clean, regularly vacuumed home is good for our mental and physical health and wellbeing. A sanitized home continually sprayed with antibacterial sprays and bleach isn't a happy and healthy home – it's a potentially toxic one. The only room that needs to be completely sterile is an operating theatre.

We don't need to routinely use anti-bac sprays and eco-unfriendly wipes in our homes. Good old soap and water cleans surfaces equally well, including killing harmful bacteria and viruses, while also being less potentially harmful for health; less likely to provoke allergic reactions; less polluting for the environment and importantly, does not contribute to the growth of superbugs or multi-strain antibiotic resistant bacteria like MRSA. When surfaces do need to be disinfected, try a 3% solution of hydrogen peroxide for a safer, more stable alternative to anti-bac sprays.

# PLANT-BASED CLOTHS AND SPONGES

All those plastic-containing, non-biodegradable, disposable cloths, wipes, brushes and sponges we buy also need to be phased out. Ideally switch to renewable, biodegradable plant-based alternatives – and do compost them where possible, rather than throwing them in the bin.

Look for wooden brushes and scourers made from plant-based materials such as cactus (also called sisal and agave) bristles or coconut fibre, which are compostable, or copper wire scourers that can be recycled. Switch polyurethane sponge-scourers for those made from loofah, cellulose or coconut fibre, and swap disposable cleaning cloths for reusable cotton rags such as old face flannels or baby muslins.

If you like paper kitchen towel for clearing up spills, bamboo paper towels can be washed several times before being composted. Cleaning wipes (like baby wipes) are a total eco no-no – switch to reusable cloths with a spray of eco-friendly cleaning product.

Microfibre cleaning cloths and "feather" dusters can be reused and they are effective at cleaning without chemicals, but every time they are used or washed, they release harmful plastic microfibres and the chemicals used to produce them into the environment, water supplies and oceans – so stick to simple cotton cloths.

To keep reusable cloths and sponges clean, cloths should be washed after each use in the washing machine, while sponges can be soaked in water and microwaved for up to 2 minutes (not metal scourers) or run through the dishwasher with your dishes on a heat-dry cycle.

# PANTRY CLEANING TRICKS

Sometimes you only need to open your kitchen cupboards to find a quick cleaning fix.

**Ketchup:** Spread a layer of ketchup (or any tomato sauce) on copper pans or brass ornaments and leave for 10 minutes, or longer if really dirty. Buff off with a soft cloth, rinse with warm water and dry thoroughly to remove dirt and tarnish.

**Banana Skins:** These are brilliant for gently cleaning and polishing plant leaves and silverware. Their potassium content means they also shine leather shoes and can buff away scuff and marks on leather upholstery too.

**Bread:** A natural alternative to a "magic eraser" product, you can use bread to remove smudges and stains from walls, wallpaper and other hard surfaces. If you have a greasy stain or spill, laying a slice of bread over it and pressing it down can help absorb all the oil and make it easier to clean.

**Olive Oil:** If you have wicker or cane furniture that needs sprucing up, take a small amount of warmed olive oil and gently rub it in with a soft cloth, ensuring it's fully absorbed. If you have stubborn burned-on food on cast-iron pans, use a drizzle of olive oil and some coarse sea salt with a stiff brush to get them clean.

**Potatoes:** Slice a potato in half and use the cut side to clean a window or mirror. Spritz the glass with water and wipe the starchy film off with a cloth for a squeaky clean. The oxalic acid in potatoes can also help break down rust, so slice a spud in half, dip it in bicarbonate of soda (baking soda) and rub it on your cast-iron pans – or any rusty implements or tools – then rinse and dry.

**Lemons:** There's a lot you can do with lemons, but they are particularly good for deodorizing stinky wooden chopping boards. Simply sprinkle the board with salt and exfoliate with the cut side of a lemon half. Let it marinate for a while, then wipe clean with a damp cloth.

For a fast and fragrant microwave clean, squeeze a lemon into 125ml (4fl oz) water in a jug, then drop the squeezed halves in too. Microwave on high power for 3–4 minutes (until the water is boiling), then leave it to stand for another 5 minutes, without opening the door. Wipe out the microwave with a clean, damp cloth and use the lemon water to scrub away any especially stubborn dried-on bits.

# LEMON AND ROSEMARY MULTIPURPOSE SPRAY

*This is a good first product to switch to as it will be in regular use in kitchens and bathrooms. I use this for most cleaning purposes, but it's not suitable for stone surfaces such as granite.*

**For a 1-litre (34fl oz) glass spray bottle**

## YOU WILL NEED

**2-3 lemon rinds**

**1-2 rosemary sprigs**

**250ml (8½fl oz) boiled water, cooled**

**250ml (8½fl oz) white vinegar**

## METHOD

Push the lemon rinds and rosemary into a glass spray bottle and pour in the cool water and vinegar.

Shake and leave to infuse for 1 week before using with a cleaning cloth.

### TIP

If you'd like to use the spray immediately, use pure essential oils instead of lemon rinds and herbs. Add 35-40 drops of your choice of essential oils to the bottle along with a dash of glycerine, then shake and spray.

## HOMEMADE ESSENTIAL OIL DIFFUSER

*For something purporting to make our homes "fresh", spray and plug-in air fresheners are among the worst offenders when it comes to indoor air pollution. Plug-ins produce a range of substances that may have harmful health effects. These toxins may be absorbed into the fabric of your home and continue to pollute the air, even after the device is un-plugged. Instead, make your own non-toxic reed diffuser to keep things fragrant, which is much more budget-friendly than store-bought diffuser sets.*

### YOU WILL NEED

**1 recycled glass bottle** (I keep and reuse the bottles from store-bought reed diffuser sets)

**100ml (3½fl oz) sweet almond oil**

**45 drops of one or two essential oils** (I love lavender and bergamot for a relaxing fragrance or peppermint and orange for something zingy)

**8 reed diffuser sticks**

### METHOD

Pour the oil into the bottle and add the essential oils.

Stand the reed sticks in the oil for a few hours, then turn the sticks upside down to ensure the oil is absorbed up the full length.

Every couple of weeks give the oil a stir and turn the sticks upside down. Replace the sticks and refresh the oils after 12 weeks or when the aroma fades.

## SIGNPOSTS

For more on:

❋ Growing your own herbs, *see* chapter 4

❋ Harmful chemicals in the home, *see* chapter 13

# 15

# INDOOR PLANTSPIRATION

"indoor plants offer two potential benefits
for us: improved psychological well-being and
improved physical human health."

Royal Horticultural Society

> **THE GOAL:**
> **TO GROW YOUR OWN INDOOR JUNGLE**

**O**N THE GREYEST OF DAYS IN WINTER OR WHEN A WORK deadline means you can't leave your desk, houseplants provide a powerful tonic. Spending time in nature is essential for wellbeing, and bringing the lush foliage of indoor plants into your home is a beautiful way to live more plantfully every day, enriching your surroundings with nourishing greenery that can help you feel calmer, be more productive and even feel happier.

There's such a quiet satisfaction to be gained from indoor growing. Getting to know each plant through the seasons, learning how to care for them, seeing them flourish – it's hugely rewarding. And people do get quite attached to their attractive house guests, with some even identifying on social media as "plant parents". While not as labour-intensive as children, of course, indoor plants do need a surprising amount of nurturing to keep them healthy and happy and even the keenest of house plant enthusiasts will have had a few casualties over the years.

It's no coincidence that the indoor growing trend has been fuelled by pandemic-related lockdowns. With people spending more time indoors away from green spaces, especially those in urban areas or without their own gardens, house plants have provided a daily "green fix" at home.

The reputed health benefits of indoor plants have been widely reported too, and people have engaged with the rather wonderful idea that their favourite spider plant might not just look beautiful but could have secret superpowers for boosting their physical and mental health. Scientific research does back up the idea that these artful arrangements are more than just a photogenic interior design trend; house plants do have a meaningful and measurable effect on health and happiness.

## A DOSE OF VITAMIN "G"

Could vitamin "G" (green) be a missing link in the human health equation? This is the question that many researchers are trying to answer, as there's a wealth of evidence to support the idea that exposure to nature contributes to improved physical and mental wellbeing, along with other established healthy habits such as staying hydrated, reducing stress levels, taking exercise and eating fruit and vegetables. Of course, eating a diet of junk food while spending lots of time in the garden isn't going to be a recipe for good health – but immersion in nature is becoming regarded as an essential building block of a healthier lifestyle, rather than just an enjoyable add-on.

Interestingly, studies have shown that even "passive engagement" with nature can be beneficial – such as looking at images of greenery or having a view of plants – and this is where house plants may have an important role to play in our homes. A study of hospital patients recovering from gallbladder surgery was the first to show that those with a view of nature from their window healed faster and needed fewer painkillers than those patients with a view of a brick wall.[1] It certainly strengthens the argument for greening up our indoor spaces, including hospitals, schools, workplaces and care homes. For those people who find it harder to spend time outdoors, whether that's through illness, disability or old age, house plants could be a simple way to help improve wellbeing.

"We are seeing significant psychological and social benefits from indoor plants," says Dr Tijana Blanusa, a plant biologist and research fellow at the University of Reading, who is also the Royal Horticultural Society's Principal Horticultural Scientist. "There's now a wealth of evidence and studies confirming that plants can improve some aspects of work productivity, workplace satisfaction and even some elements of stress. One of our own studies revealed significant positive effects of plants in offices and break-out spaces on perceived, self-reported attention, efficiency, creativity, productivity and stress reduction.[2] Plants do have a role to play in terms of improving quality of life, especially in environments such as offices and schools – plus people just really enjoy being surrounded by plants."

Dr Blanusa recalls a situation that reveals just how attached people can become to plants in their environment, when after completing a study in an office space, her team removed the plants used for the experiment and the employees demanded the company reinstated the greenery. "It was very interesting to see how taking away the plants aroused such strong feelings, although that wasn't part of the study," she says. "We know there are significant psychological benefits in having indoor greenery, but it could also be that when people are surrounded by plants, they perceive the air quality to be better, they feel healthier, less stressed and are consequently more productive and happier in their work – so even without actually doing anything, just by being there the plants are beneficial."

So how can we all incorporate the benefits of biophilic design – the concept of increasing our connectivity with the natural environment in architecture and interior design – in our own homes? Introducing a mix of shapes, sizes and colours of plants in the home has been shown to positively influence productivity and wellbeing, and even some physical responses such as pulse rate, so if you work from home, popping some plants in your home office could help you achieve more and reduce your stress levels.

We may not yet fully understand the full picture of how plants can improve our mental and physical wellbeing, but it's clear that filling our homes and workspaces with houseplants is a win all round. Experts also recommend improving the view from your windows as a tonic for days when you have to spend a lot of time indoors, so if your kitchen window looks out onto a bare wall, for example, consider planting a green wall or using climbing plants in containers to add greenery. You can plant up window boxes, arrange pots on balconies or in front of patio doors – anything you can do to ensure your windows frame views of lush green foliage and flowers as much as possible.

## CREATING A CLEAN AIR ZONE

Plants have been widely touted as natural air purifiers, with many associated with specific benefits. For example, having English ivy (*Hedera helix*) in the bathroom is often said to help reduce airborne faecal particles and mould, whereas orchids and succulents are reputedly good for oxygenating bedrooms during the night, although many popularly quoted claims of this nature are often unsubstantiated by the science. While scientists are actively exploring if houseplants could be acting as living air purifiers in our homes, the latest research suggests that their air filtering powers may have been a little overstated.

When we think of air pollution, we typically think of outdoor sources such as car exhaust fumes and factory emissions, but increasingly, air pollution is not just a problem outdoors. Studies have found that indoor air can be two to five times as polluted as outdoor air, with over a third of the emissions coming from chemicals in products such as cleaning sprays, deodorant, paint, carpets and, ironically, air fresheners,[3] some of which may be harmful to health.

We know that trees and shrubs can trap harmful particulate pollution, helping to keep the air cleaner in gardens and outdoor spaces, although their impact depends on a variety of factors such as wind direction, humidity levels and canopy density, which is why the best solution for cleaner air is always to reduce pollution at the source.[4] Trees of course play a vital role in removing carbon dioxide from the atmosphere and replenishing oxygen. In Chapter 1 (page 17), we discovered why walking in the forest offers the most powerful breath of fresh air of all. Knowing this, it would make sense that house plants may play a similar role indoors. But many of the current claims made for house plants as air purifiers are founded on The Clean Air Study undertaken by NASA in 1989, which showed that plants can filter not only carbon dioxide but also a range of harmful household compounds, including benzene (in paint and detergents), formaldehyde (used in products such as laminate flooring and paper towels) and ammonia (cleaning products).

It's important to look at this research in context, according to Dr Blanusa. "We know plants indoors are capable of filtering compounds from the air, and the more controlled the environment the bigger the effect, but we are now re-evaluating the studies from the late 80s and the NASA study, because we have to consider the scale and environmental conditions of those experiments," she explains.

Put simply, the experiments were not based on real-life levels of contamination, because the resolution of the instruments used back then couldn't pick up the small readings that scientists can detect today, which meant they had to expose plants to levels of a compound that would never be found in a real home.

"What scientists now are trying to discover is if plants uptake those compounds at the same rate when the levels are reduced to conditions found in a typical home," says Dr Blanusa. "It may be that under such high exposure the plant's reaction and uptake is much greater than it would be under normal levels of exposure."

Carbon uptake rates are generally much lower in indoor plants than in outdoor plants, and probably too low to make much difference to air quality in a room-size space, mainly because of the lack of light indoors. Light makes a plant grow more actively and uptake higher levels of carbon dioxide, so to make any appreciable difference to carbon levels in your living room, you'd need an exceptionally light-filled space and at least five actively growing plants.[5]

However, there are some substances that even at very low concentrations in the air can be very harmful for human health, and if plants are proven to filter these out even in tiny amounts, this could make a big difference to health.

In the meantime, while plants may not be the panacea of pollution control in our homes, if you combine abundant plant parenting with other measures such as regularly opening windows (unless you live close to heavy traffic or industry) and reducing the potential pollutants coming into your home in DIY materials and cleaning products, you can enjoy a cleaner, greener home.

## GROWING YOUR OWN INDOOR JUNGLE

By now, you're hopefully sold on the many benefits of indoor growing – but be warned: house plants can be fickle characters. One minute they look lush and vibrant in the garden centre, but after a few months in your home they have drooped, wilted and developed crispy brown leaves. It's not that house plants are necessarily fussier than any other plants; but because they are kept indoors in a pot, they are entirely dependent on you and your home to provide everything they need, and we don't always fully understand how to meet those needs. However, location, location, location is the key.

"Always buy a plant based on the conditions of the area in which you want to place it," says Rob Stirling, horticultural advisor for the RHS. "They are living plants first and ornaments second, and they are at much higher risk of failure if you treat them as just an ornament."

While indoor plants are usually chosen for their decorative, often sculptural, beauty, it's wasteful of planetary resources – and your own hard-earned money – to buy plants and just hope they will thrive where you want them to live, rather than where they will be happiest, because they probably won't survive for long. So always check the care label or look up the requirements of your new house guest to discover where they will feel most at home.

"Many house plants are native to tropical countries, where conditions would be very different to those found in the average house in the UK or USA," says Rob. "One of the main issues is low humidity. The average humidity indoors probably equates to the humidity found in a desert, usually around 20–30%, especially when central heating is on in the winter. Consequently, when you want to grow plants that come from the tropics, potentially even rainforest regions, people often find the edges of the foliage goes brown. It's an indication that the plant is suffering from water stress and often it's a humidity rather than a watering issue."

# HOW TO HAVE HEALTHY, HAPPY HOUSEPLANTS

## PUT THE RIGHT PLANT IN THE RIGHT LOCATION

Always choose a plant that suits where you want to put it. For example, bathrooms often don't have very good light – windows may be small and are usually frosted – so any bathroom plants will need to be shade tolerant and happy with humidity, such as tropical ferns. A brighter room with plenty of natural daylight will provide a happy home for many varieties, from monstera to fiddle-leaf fig, while sun-loving plants such as money plants or desert varieties such as aloe vera will be happy in direct sunlight.

## GROW IN GROUPS

Creating lush groups of plants doesn't just look good for photoshoots or Instagram posts, the microclimate created by the group helps the plants stay healthy. Just like in a real jungle or forest, plants support each other by releasing moisture through transpiration from their leaves and creating their own microclimate. Location is still important, however. For example, if you group cacti in a shady position, they won't be happy, so look for plants that all require a similar position and growing conditions, so they all thrive equally.

## ONLY WATER WHEN THEY NEED IT

Rather than watering routinely, it's best to check routinely – check if the soil is dry on the surface, and if you push your finger into the soil about an inch and it feels damp, don't water it, just check again a few days later. Only water when the plants need it, not when it fits into your routine or you may end up with root rot.

## PUT A STOP TO THE ROT

Plants should always be able to drain excess water – so either keep the plant in its original plastic pot on top of some gravel inside an exterior pot (the inner pot should have holes in the base) or use a pot with holes on the base placed on a saucer or tray. Putting pebbles or leca in the bottom of a pot is a good way to keep it well drained and help it thrive. You can also mix leca balls into the potting compost.

## KEEP AN EYE ON HUMIDITY

One solution to the low humidity in many homes is to stand your plant on a saucer over a tray filled with wet gravel or leca balls (baked clay balls). The moisture this creates around the plant will help.

## ONLY FEED A HEALTHY, ACTIVELY GROWING PLANT

This seems counter-intuitive because we are encouraged to eat nourishing food when we are sick. But plants use food very differently to us, and fertilizer is not the be-all and end-all of their nutrition. "Plants create sugars from daylight, which they then use as fuel to process fertilizer," explains Rob. "If the plant is sick, losing its leaves and not photosynthesizing very well, it won't be creating that sugar from sunlight, which means it can't process the fertilizer. This is why, if you give food to a sick plant it can make it worse." This is also the reason you should take a break from feeding in the winter months, when plants are not growing so actively. Some plants, such as orchids, don't really need much feeding at all.

## POT SIZE IS IMPORTANT

If the plant looks as though it's in a very small pot for its size, then it's a good idea to repot. Not into a huge pot, just the next size up. In a large pot, there's a danger the soil will stay wet for too long after watering, as when the pot is too big for the root ball it can't absorb the water quickly enough and this leads to root rot. Some plants don't like root disturbance, so always check the care labels before repotting.

## USE THE RIGHT COMPOST

Never use ordinary garden compost for house plants as this can be naturally full of bacteria and fungi that comes from the decomposing process and it may introduce pathogens to your houseplants – which is riskier to plant health in the confines of a pot than in the ground outside. A specialist potting mix will be free of these pathogens.

## GIVE THEM A CLEAN

Wiping dust off plant leaves with a damp cloth not only keeps them looking lovely, it also helps them breathe better and absorb more light, fuelling their growth.

## MAKE PLANT RETIREMENT PLANS

Sadly, plants don't last forever, and as they age their metabolism slows, often in response to lower light levels in your home compared to the nursery they were grown in. As your plants age and become less active, add more plants to your collection to boost their benefits.

# ARE HOUSE PLANTS ECO-FRIENDLY?

## PLANT MILES AND CARBON FOOTPRINT

Although most varieties of houseplants are native to tropical and desert regions from South America to Africa and south-east Asia, they are cultivated for supply to garden centres so our love of indoor plants is not usually damaging local biodiversity. In the UK, for example, most house plants are grown and propagated commercially in a more sustainable way either in the UK or European countries such as the Netherlands, which means they are not usually being transported thousands of miles, although energy may be used to heat greenhouses and there's water usage to factor in too.

# WHICH HOUSE PLANTS GROW BEST WHERE?

Always choose a plant you love that will also be happy in your chosen location. Some plants are more tolerant than others and will cope in a variety of conditions; others are fussier about where they live, so always check the care instructions.

**Indirect sunlight:** Swiss cheese plants *(Monstera deliciosa)*, ferns, areca palm *(Dypsis lutescens)*, calathea *(Calathea orbifolia)*

**Bright, but not direct sunlight:** Chinese money plant *(Pilea peperomioides)*, false shamrock *(Oxalis triangularis)*, fiddle-leaf fig *(Ficus lyrata)*, golden pothos or devil's ivy *(Epipremnum aureum)*, rubber plant *(Ficus elastica)*

**Direct sunlight:** aloe vera, cacti, spineless yucca *(Yucca elephantipes)*, money or jade plant *(Crassula ovata)*, mother-in-law's tongue *(Sansevieria trifasciata)*

**Shade or half-shade:** succulents, mother-in-law's tongue *(Sansevieria trifasciata)*, emerald palm *(Zamioculcas zamiifolia)*, spider plant *(chlorophytum comosum)*, peace lilies *(Spathiphyllum Wallisii)*

However, as the trend for house plants grows, even importing from relatively nearby countries still racks up a lot of plant miles. On the other hand, growing plants in naturally hotter climates further afield could reduce the need for heated greenhouses that are required for growing in a cooler climate.

As with all things related to carbon footprint, it's a bit of a minefield to untangle the best options, especially with so many variables to consider. In time, it would be good to see suppliers required to label their plants so consumers can see the carbon footprint of their potential purchases. The best way for you to help is to take good care of your plants to give them a long, healthy life so they don't need to be replaced every few months.

## PLASTIC POTS

In the UK alone, 500 million plastic seed trays and plant pots are used by gardeners every year, and they are rarely recycled. Look for biodegradable or ceramic pots, buy from garden centres that offer a recycling scheme for returned pots or keep them to reuse again in your garden.

Avoiding "single use" plants, such as poinsettias grown for Christmas, can also reduce the waste of planetary resources; opt instead for seasonal varieties that can be kept to bloom again the next year or planted out in the garden after flowering, such as spring bulbs.

## PEAT-FREE COMPOST

Many houseplants are grown in peat-based compost, even if they are switched to peat-free by retailers. You can help by always using peat-free potting mixes and supporting garden centres, nurseries and mail order suppliers that also use peat-free soil, ideally throughout the growing process.

# IS HOUSE-PLANT FOOD VEGAN-FRIENDLY?

From dried blood to bone meal or fish scales, the ingredients in houseplant fertilizers are often derived from animal ingredients. However, it's possible to find more organic and plant-based houseplant feeds these days. Some plant-based varieties use seaweed – but do ensure you buy a brand using sustainably harvested seaweed.

Simple plant foods from your pantry include chopped, dried banana peel, buried in the compost, which will gradually release minerals; and the cooled cooking water from boiling vegetables.

# HOUSE PLANTS VS CUT FLOWERS

While house plants certainly have an environmental impact, if well cared for, they can thrive happily in your home for several years. Not so cut flowers, which will last for around a week or so. Cut flowers grown organically in your garden have a carbon footprint of zero, while a bouquet of imported blooms could have a substantial footprint of around 30kg (66lbs) $CO_2e$ (based on flowers imported to the UK from countries such as the Netherlands and Kenya). If you regularly buy a bunch of flowers when you go shopping, this could potentially be the highest carbon-producing item in your trolley.

House plants are certainly an eco-friendlier way to bring nature into your home or for giving as gifts, but when only a bouquet will do, try to buy in-season, locally grown blooms wherever possible, as one bunch of mixed varieties grown outdoors in the UK and sold locally, will produce just 1.7kg (3½lbs) $CO_2e$.[6]

## PLANTS FOR FREE

The most sustainable way to build your houseplant collection is by not buying plants at all. Instead, try plant exchanges, growing them from seed or taking cuttings and suckers – which are not only more sustainable methods of growing, but also cost nothing. It's usually best to grow plants from seed or cuttings in spring and summer, when plants are more naturally active.

## AVOCADO EXPERIMENT

Probably thanks to our obsession with avocados, the *Persea americana* plant is also becoming popular as a houseplant. Plus, it's really fun to grow from seed. Simply wash an avocado stone clean and stick 4 pins or toothpicks horizontally into the narrower end of the stone at 12, 3, 6 and 9 o'clock, about 2cm (¾in) from the top. The idea is to create supports to rest on the rim of a small jar of water, so the base of the avocado stone is under water. Pop the glass in a very sunny spot and change the water regularly to avoid mould forming. After a few weeks, you should see a split in the base and roots will emerge, followed by a shoot from the top a few weeks later. Once your shoot reaches around 20cm (8in), remove the pins/sticks and put it in a pot with drainage holes with some potting compost, leaving the top of the stone jutting slightly out of the compost. Keep it moist and wait for large oval leaves to appear.

Sadly, you probably won't be harvesting avocados any time soon, because avocados have a complex pollination process to produce fruit, but it's still an attractive plant to grow.

## STEM CUTTINGS

A stem cutting is so easy to do. Simply cut off a branch of the plant using secateurs, just below a node (bump) in the stem, then strip off the lower leaves. Pop the cutting in a clear glass or bottle with some water and replace it weekly. Within a few weeks you should see the cutting developing roots, and once a good root system is established, you can pot it up with potting compost. Pinch out the tips of the plant to encourage it to branch out. Many types of house plants can be grown from cuttings, including rubber plants, African violets, coleus, ivy, epipremnum (such as devil's ivy and golden pothos), scented geraniums, and *Philodrendron scandens*. This technique works with most fast-growing houseplants with multiple stems, but if you're not sure if it will work with your plant – just have a go, it really can't hurt to try it.

## SUCCULENTS

These fleshy, thick-leaved sculptural plants are very popular, and they are also easy to take cuttings from. Fill a pot with seed and cactus compost (this has more added sand to make it more free-draining than potting compost) and give it a water. Using a clean, sharp knife (or remove gently by hand if they come off easily) remove a leaf from the base of the plant, and place on the pot, allowing the cut edge to touch the compost. Keep it moist by spraying it with water every few days and, after around a month, you should notice small roots forming, which then turn into small rosettes of new leaves. Carefully transfer to larger pots and watch them grow.

## DIVIDE AND CONQUER

Many houseplants can be split, or divided into sections and repotted to create new plants for free. These plants have a sturdy ball of roots at the base of several stems, and you can usually tell when they are ready as they will start to look too big for their pot or roots may start trying to escape. To divide them, just carefully remove the plant from its pot, tease apart the root ball and using a sharp knife split the clump into sections, ensuring each one has a good-sized portion of root and leaves. Pot up individually in fresh potting compost. Plants with which to try this technique are peace lilies, asparagus fern, snake plant, Boston fern and philodendron. Plants like aloe vera produce offshoots from the root that can be easily divided and re-potted, while Chinese money plants (*Pilea peperomioides*) produce suckers that can be gently cut off the main root (just dig down carefully) and will grow roots in a glass of water using the stem-cutting technique above.

## SIGNPOSTS

For more on:

- 🌿 Nature and wellbeing, *see* chapter 1
- 🌿 Peat-free compost, *see* chapter 3
- 🌿 Eco-friendly gardening, *see* chapter 5
- 🌿 Harmful chemicals in the home, *see* chapters 13 and 14

# CONCLUSION

Now you've reached the end of this book, my hope is that you feel inspired to infuse every aspect of your life with plant powers – and have fun doing it. If I've learned anything on my own continually evolving journey to "living plantfully", it often means breaking a few "rules" and not being afraid to do things a little differently. Being brave about letting go of old habits and traditions and establishing new, more positive ones will enhance your life in so many ways, and may have a wider impact too. Not everyone will agree with the idea of letting weeds grow wild, serving roasted squash for Sunday lunch or using vinegar to scrub the bathroom, but – as the saying goes – you do you.

Throughout this book I've advocated a gentle, holistic approach to living plantfully, because you should feel excited about trying something new, not pressured or daunted. There's no need to become a strict vegan overnight, turn your whole backyard into a veg plot or throw away every product in your cleaning cupboard – even if these things are your ultimate goal – because most experts agree that making gradual, achievable changes is by far the best way to stick to them in the long term. While some new habits take time to become fully ingrained, there are plenty of ideas in this book that you can put into practice immediately, which cost almost nothing to do. I'm sure if you looked in your fridge right now you could find the ingredients to put together a delicious meat-free meal, even without going shopping. Alternatively, you could clear your head – and get a beneficial dose of healthy bacteria – by popping into the garden and getting your hands dirty or heading out for a walk in a local green space. Living plantfully can be as simple as putting your shoes on and going outside.

The messages around what we should eat and how we should live can sometimes be confusing and contradictory, but every reputable health professional, environmentalist and scientist agrees that eating a diverse range of whole plant foods and connecting with nature are the number one ways to boost our physical and mental health, while also giving the planet its best chance of survival. For every meal you prepare, every lifestyle decision you make or product you buy, think about how to make it more plantful first and you'll not only be enriching your own wellbeing but also that of the global community and the Earth we share.

By now, I hope you are excited about embracing a more joyful, nourishing and sustainable way of living, so I'll simply conclude this labour of love by reminding you of the core idea that sparked this book in the first place: *everything that is naturally good for us is good for the planet.*

Fill your home, your plate and your life with plants, spend more time in nature and make deeper connections with the wild world around you, and you too will flourish like a rogue dandelion on an unmown lawn in spring.

# ACKNOWLEDGEMENTS

With huge thanks to my family for patiently bearing with me during the writing of this book; to my parents, for all their love and support over the years; to my agent Clare Grist Taylor for spotting the potential in this book and being incredibly supportive throughout the process; to my publisher Jo Lal, editor Beth Bishop and the team at Welbeck Balance for getting behind the Living Plantfully concept and working with me to create a beautiful book; and to all my lovely friends and colleagues who have cheered me on in their own wonderful ways.

I have had the pleasure of talking to many colleagues, friends and contributing experts during the writing of this book and the creation of resources for www.livingplantfully.co.uk, who have kindly shared their incredible insight and expertise. I'd like to thank the following people and organizations for their wisdom.

Jess Arnaudin, plant-based beauty expert and author, jessarnaudin.com
Dr Rupy Aujla, founder of The Doctor's Kitchen, thedoctorskitchen.com
Anita Bean, registered nutritionist and author, anitabean.co.uk
Dr Tijana Blanusa, University of Reading and the Royal Horticultural Society, rhs.org.uk
Helen Bostock, Royal Horticultural Society, rhs.org.uk
John Cherry, regenerative farmer and founder of Groundswell, groundswellag.com
Sonja Dibbin, founder of Adore Your Outdoors, adoreyouroutdoors.co.uk
Jen Gale, founder of Sustainable(ish), asustainablelife.co.uk
Azmina Govindji, dietitian and media nutritionist, azminanutrition.com
Wendy Graham, author and blogger, moralfibres.co.uk
Judith Hann, TV presenter, author and herb expert
Russell Horsey, chartered arboriculturalist, woodlanddwelling.co.uk
Tom Hunt, chef and author, tomsfeast.com
Anna Jones, author and food writer, annajones.co.uk
Dr Shireen Kassam, founder and director of Plant-Based Health Professionals, plantbasedhealthprofessionals.com

Beth Kempton, author and founder of Do What You Love, bethkempton.com

Josiah Meldrum, co-founder of Hodmedod, producers of ancient grains and pulses, hodmedods.co.uk

Adele Nozedar, expert forager, founder of Brecon Beacons Foraging and author, breconbeaconsforaging.com

Micaela Sharp, TV presenter and interior designer, micaelasharpdesign.com

Sarah Shorley, Urban Tree Team, Woodland Trust, woodlandtrust.org.uk

Lisa Simon, registered dietitian, plantbasedhealthonline.com

Lucy Hutchings, gardener, author and founder of She Grows Veg, shegrowsveg.com

Rob Stirling, Royal Horticultural Society, rhs.org.uk

Helen White, special advisor on household waste at wrap.org.uk

Alice Whitehead, writer, allotmenteer and founder of Save Our Street Trees, saveourstreettrees.org

Emily Wysock-Wright, wellbeing expert and founder of Energetically Emily, energeticallyemily.com

# FURTHER READING

## SOME OF MY FAVOURITE BOOKS
## ON PLANT-BASED FOOD AND NUTRITION

*15-Minute Vegan* by Katy Beskow (Quadrille, 2017)

*Be More Vegan* by Niki Webster (Welbeck, 2020)

*Doctor's Kitchen 3-2-1* by Dr Rupy Aujla (Thorsons, 2020)

*Eat Green* by Melissa Hemsley (Ebury Press, 2020)

*Eat More, Live Well* by Dr Megan Rossi (Penguin Life, 2021)

*Eat to Save the Planet* by Annie Bell (One Boat, 2020)

*Eating for Pleasure, People and & Planet* by Tom Hunt (Kyle Books, 2020)

*The Green Roasting Tin* by Rukmini Iyer (Square Peg, 2018)

*One Pot, Pan, Planet* by Anna Jones (Fourth Estate, 2021)

*The Part-Time Vegetarian* by Nicola Graimes (Nourish Books, 2015)

*Speedy BOSH!* By Henry Firth and Ian Theasby (HQ, 2020)

*Vegan Savvy* by Azmina Govindji (Pavilion, 2020)

*Vegetarian Meals in 30 Minutes* by Anita Bean (Bloomsbury Sport, 2019)

## ALSO WELL WORTH A READ

### FORAGING AND WILD FOODS

*The Hedgerow Handbook: Recipe, Remedies and Rituals* by Adele Nozedar (Square Peg, 2012)

*Food for Free* by Richard Mabey (Collins, new edition, 2012)

*The Forager's Calendar* by John Wright (Profile Books, 2020)

### NATURE

*The Garden Jungle* by Dave Goulson (Jonathan Cape, 2019)

*The Hidden Life of Trees* by Peter Wohlleben (William Collins Books, 2017)

*Nature Cure* by Richard Mabey (Vintage, 2008)

### GROWING

*A Pocketful of Herbs* by Jekka McVicar (Bloomsbury Absolute, 2019)

*The Art of Mindful Gardening* by Ark Redwood (Leaping Hare/Ivy Press, 2011)

*Eat What You Grow* by Alys Fowler (Kyle Books, 2021)
*Get Up and Grow* by Lucy Hutchings (Hardie Grant, 2021)
*Herbs* by Judith Hann (Nourish Books, 2017)

## LIVING WELL
*How to Live* by Professor Robert Thomas (Short Books, 2020)
*Spoon-Fed* by Tim Spector (Vintage, 2022)

## SUSTAINABILITY
*How Bad Are Bananas?* by Mike Berners-Lee (Profile Books, 2020)
*Is it Really Green?* By Georgina Wilson-Powell (DK, 2021)
*The Sustainable(ish) Living Guide* by Jen Gale (Green Tree, 2020)

## HOME
*Fresh, Clean Home* by Wendy Graham (Pavilion, 2018)
*Plant-Based Beauty* by Jess Arnaudin (Aster, 2019)
*Slow Death by Rubber Duck* by Rick Smith and Bruce Lourie
(Counterpoint, 2011)

# REFERENCES

**INTRODUCTION**

1. Xu, X. et al. 2021. "Global Greenhouse Gas Emissions from Animal-Based Foods Are Twice Those of Plant-Based Foods," Nature Food 2(9): 724–32.

2. Springmann, M. et al. 2018. "Options for Keeping the Food System within Environmental Limits," Nature 562(7728): 519–25.

3. Alexandratos, N, Bruinsma, J, "World Agriculture Towards 2030/2050," 2012 Revision, Food and Agriculture Organization of the United Nations, viewed 20 January 2022, <https://www.fao.org/3/ap106e/ap106e.pdf>

**CHAPTER 1**

1. Gladwell VF, Brown DK, Wood C, Sandercock GR, Barton JL. The great outdoors: how a green exercise environment can benefit all. Extrem Physiol Med. 2013;2(1):3. Published 2013 Jan 3. doi:10.1186/2046-7648-2-3

2. Selway CA, Mills JG, Weinstein P, Skelly C, Yadav S, Lowe A, Breed MF, Weyrich LS, 2020. "Transfer of environmental microbes to the skin and respiratory tract of humans after urban green space exposure," Environ Int. Dec;145, vdoi: 10.1016/j.envint.2020.106084

3. Dimitrov, S, Hulteng E, Hong S, 2017. "Inflammation and exercise: Inhibition of monocytic intracellular TNF production by acute exercise via β2-adrenergic activation," Brain, Behavior, and Immunity:61: 60–68, viewed 20 January 2022, <www.sciencedirect.com/science/article/pii/S0889159116305645>

4. White, M.P., Alcock, I., Grellier, J. et al. Spending at least 120 minutes a week in nature is associated with good health and wellbeing. Sci Rep 9, 7730 (2019), viewed 20 January 2022, <doi.org/10.1038/ s41598-019-44097-3>

5. Saraev, V, O'Brien, L, Valatin, G, Bursnell, M, "Valuing the mental health benefits of woodlands," 2021, Forest Research, viewed 20 January 2022, <www.forestresearch.gov.uk/documents/8217/FRRP034.pdf>

6. Weiler, N, "Awe Walks Boost Emotional Well-being", 2020, University of California San Francisco, viewed 20 January 2022, <www.ucsf.edu/news/2020/09/418551/awe-walks-boost-emotional-well-being>

**CHAPTER 2**

1. Harrad, L, "A Prescription for Good Health," 2021, Living Plantfully, viewed 20 January 2022, <livingplantfully.co.uk/feature/a-prescription-for-good-health/>

2. Pandey, KB, Rizvi, SI, "Plant polyphenols as dietary antioxidants in human health and disease", 2009, US National Library of Medicine National Institutes of Health, viewed 20 January 2022, <www.ncbi.nlm.nih.gov/pmc/articles/PMC2835915/>

3.  EAT, "Healthy Diets from Sustainable Food Systems – A Summary Report of the Eat-Lancet Commission," 2019, EAT, viewed 20 January 2022, <eatforum.org/content/uploads/2019/07/EAT-Lancet_Commission_Summary_ Report.pdf>

4.  United Nations Framework Convention on Climate Change, "What is the Paris Agreement?", 2021, United Nations Framework Convention on Climate Change, viewed 20 January 2022, <unfccc.int/process-and-meetings/the-paris-agreement/the-paris-agreement>

5.  Knüppel, A, Papier, K, Fensom, G K, Appleby, P N, Schmidt, J A, Tong, T Y N, Travis, R C, Key, T J, Perez-Cornago, A, "Meat intake and cancer risk: Prospective analyses in UK Biobank," 2020, International Journal of Epidemiology 49 (5), viewed 20 January 2022, <academic.oup.com/ije/article/49/5/1540/5894731?login=true>

6.  Papier, K, Fensom, G K, Knüppel, A, Appleby, P N, Schmidt, J A, Tong, T Y N, Travis, R C, Key, T J, Perez-Cornago, A, "*Meat consumption and risk of 25 common conditions: outcome-wide analyses in 475,000 men and women in the UK Biobank study*," 2021, BMC Medicine, viewed 20 January 2022, <bmcmedicine.biomedcentral.com/articles/10.1186/s12916-021-01922-9>

7.  Ritchie, H, "Half of the world's habitable land is used for agriculture," 2019, Our World in Data, viewed 20 January 2022, <ourworldindata.org/global-land-for-agriculture>

8.  Kew Gardens, State of the World's Plants and Fungi report, 2020

9.  Sutcliffe C, Hess T, "*The global avocado crisis and resilience in the UK's fresh fruit and vegetable supply system*," 2017, Global Food Security, viewed 20 January 2022, <www.foodsecurity.ac.uk/blog/global-avocado-crisis-resilience-uks-fresh-fruit-vegetable-supply-system/>

## CHAPTER 3

1.  Blum, W E H, Zechmeister-Boltenstern S, Keiblinger K M, "*Does Soil Contribute to the Human Gut Microbiome?*" 2019, National Library of Medicine National Institutes of Health, viewed 20 January 2022, <www.ncbi.nlm.nih.gov/pmc/articles/PMC6780873/>

2.  Tester-Jones, M., White, M.P., Elliott, L.R. et al. Results from an 18-country cross-sectional study examining experiences of nature for people with common mental health disorders. Sci Rep 10, 19408 (2020). <doi.org/10.1038/s41598-020-75825-9>

3.  Schlanger, Z, "*Dirt has a microbiome, and it may double as an antidepressant*," 2017, Quartz, viewed 20 January 2022, <qz.com/993258/dirt-has-a-microbiome-and-it-may-double-as-an-antidepressant/>

4.  Olafsdottir, G, Cloke, P, Lin, J, "Green exercise is associated with better cell aging profiles," 2016, The European Journal of Public Health, viewed 20 January 2022, <www.researchgate.net/publication/311695511_Green_exercise_is_associated_with_ better_cell_aging_profiles>

5.  Horton, H, "*Cocktail of pesticides in almost all oranges and grapes, UK study finds*," 2021, The Guardian, viewed 20 January 2022, <www.theguardian.com/environment/2021/sep/29/cocktail-pesticides-almost-all-oranges-grapes-uk-study>

6.  WRAP, "Developing a sustainable food system," 2021, WRAP, viewed 20 January 2022, <wrap.org.uk/taking-action/food-drink274>

7.   Roberts, J, "Growing the green economy – in your back garden," 2018, Green Economy Coalition, viewed 20 January 2022, <www.greeneconomycoalition.org/news-and-resources/how-to-grow-the-green-economy-in-your-back-garden>

8.  Royal Horticultural Society, "10 ways to be more sustainable in your garden," 2021, Royal Horticultural Society, viewed 20 January 2022, <www.rhs.org.uk/advice/gardening-for-the-environment/planet-friendly-gardening-tips>

9.  Royal Horticultural Society, "Peat-free gardening," 2021, Royal Horticultural Society, viewed 20 January 2022, <www.rhs.org.uk/advice/peat>

10. Fofaria, N M, Srivastava, S K, "Mechanism of the anticancer effect of phytochemicals," 2015, The Enzymes; and Pradhan N, Patra, S K, "Epigenetic dietary interventions for prevention of cancer," 2019, Epigenetics of Cancer Prevention, viewed 20 January 2022, <www.sciencedirect.com/topics/medicine-and-dentistry/sulforaphane>

**CHAPTER 5**

1.  United Nations, "68% of the world population projected to live in urban areas by 2050," 2018, United Nations, viewed 20 January 2022, <www.un.org/development/desa/en/news/population/2018-revision-of-world-urbanization-prospects.html>

2.  Plantlife, "*No Mow May: how to get ten times more bees on your lockdown lawn*," 2021, Plantlife, viewed 20 January 2022, <www.plantlife.org.uk/uk/about-us/news/no-mow-may-how-to-get-ten-times-more-bees-on-your-lockdown-lawn>

3.  State of the World's Plants and Fungi report, 2020

4.  State of the World's Plants and Fungi report, 2020

5.  Salisbury A, Bostock H, et al, "Plants for Bugs: *does the geographical origin of plants affect the abundance and diversity of the invertebrates they support?*", 2019, Royal Horticultural Society, viewed 20 January 2022, <www.rhs.org.uk/science/conservation-biodiversity/plants-for-bugs>

6.  Benjamin B. Phillips, Anila Navaratnam, Joel Hooper, James M. Bullock, Juliet L. Osborne, Kevin J. Gaston, "Road verge extent and habitat composition across Great Britain", Landscape and Urban Planning, Volume 214, 2021, 104159,ISSN 0169-2046, <doi.org/10.1016/j.landurbplan.2021.104159>, <www.sciencedirect.com/science/article/pii/S0169204621001225>

7.  Royal Horticultural Society, "Gardening Matters: Front Gardens," 2021, Royal Horticultural Society, viewed 20 January 2022, <www.rhs.org.uk/science/pdf/Gardening-matters-Front-Gardens-urban-greening.pdf>

**CHAPTER 6**

1.  Carvalho, M.R, Jaramillo, C, De La Parra, F, Caballero-Rodríguez, D, Herrera, F, Wing, S, Turner, B.L, D'Apolito, C, Romero-Báez, M, Silvestro, D, et al, "*Extinction at the end-Cretaceous and the origin of modern Neotropical rainforests,*" 2021, Science, vol. 372, issue 6537, viewed 20 January 2022, <www.science.org/doi/10.1126/science.abf1969>

2. Crowther, T. W., Glick, H. B., Covey, K. R., Bettigole, C., Maynard, D. S., Thomas, S. M., & Tuanmu, M. N. (2015). "Mapping tree density at a global scale". Nature, 525(7568), 201-205.

3. Ritchie, H, Roser, M, "Forests and Deforestation," 2021, Our World in Data, viewed 20 January 2022, <https://ourworldindata.org/deforestation>

4. Schwartz, J, "11 of the world's most threatened forests," 2015, World Wide Fund for Nature, viewed 20 January 2020, <www.worldwildlife.org/stories/11-of-the-world-s-most-threatened-forests>

5. Johnson, H.J, "Rainforest', 2015, National Geographic, viewed 20 January 2022, <www.nationalgeographic.org/encyclopedia/rain-forest/>

6. World Wide Fund for Nature, "Amazon," 2021, World Wide Fund for Nature, viewed 20 January 2022, <www.worldwildlife.org/places/amazon>

7. Chester Zoo, "What is palm oil," 2021, Chester Zoo, viewed 20 January 2022, <www.chesterzoo.org/what-you-can-do/our-campaigns/sustainable-palm-oil/what-is-palm-oil/>

8. World Wide Fund for Nature, "8 things to know about palm oil," 2021, World Wide Fund for Nature, viewed 20 January 2022, <www.wwf.org.uk/updates/8-things-know-about-palm-oil>

9. Paul Tullis, "How the world got hooked on palm oil," 2019, The Guardian, viewed 20 January 2022, <www.theguardian.com/news/2019/feb/19/palm-oil-ingredient-biscuits-shampoo-environmental>

10. World Wide Fund for Nature, "Are brands committed to a responsible palm oil future," 2021, World Wide Fund for Nature, viewed 20 January 2022, <palmoilscorecard.panda.org/#/home>

11. Chester Zoo, "Sustainable palm oil shopping list," 2021, Chester Zoo, viewed 20 January 2022, <www.chesterzoo.org/schools/resources/sustainable-palm-oil-shopping-list/>

12. Berners-Lees, M. (2020). How Bad Are Bananas. (rev. ed.), London: Profile Books.

13. Alvarsson et al. "Stress Recovery during Exposure to Nature Sound and Environmental Noise", International Journal of Environmental Research and Public Health, 2010.

14. Office for National Statistics, "UK air pollution removal: how much pollution does vegetation remove in your area?" 2018, Office for National Statistics, viewed 20 January 2022, <www.ons.gov.uk/economy/environmentalaccounts/articles/ukairpollutionremovalhowmuchpollutiondoesvegetationremoveinyourarea/2018-07-30>

15. Ready, R, Diffendal, T, Gallion B, Mussenden, S, "The Role of Trees," 2019, University of Maryland's Howard Center for Investigative Journalism, viewed 20 January 2022, <cnsmaryland.org/interactives/summer-2019/code-red/role-of-trees.html>

16. Baltimore Tree Trust, "Our Story", 2021, Baltimore Tree Trust, viewed 20 January 2022, <www.baltimoretreetrust.org/about-us/our-story/>

17. ETH Zürich, "Predicting climate change: *Understanding carbon cycle feedbacks to predict climate change at large scale,*" 2019, American Association for the Advancement of Science, viewed 20 January 2022, <www.eurekalert.org/news-releases/557130>

**CHAPTER 7**

1. The LEAP Project (Livestock, Environment and People), Oxford University

2. Stewart, H, Hyman, J, "Americans Still Can Meet Fruit and Vegetable Dietary Guidelines for $2.10-$2.60 per Day," 2019, US Department of Agriculture Economic Research Service, viewed 20 January 2022, <www.ers.usda.gov/amber-waves/2019/june/americans-still-can-meet-fruit-and-vegetable-dietary-guidelines-for-210-260-per-day/275>

3. Rauber, F, da Costa Louzada, M.L, Steele, E.M, Millett, C, Monteiro, C.A, Levy, R.B, *"Ultra-Processed Food Consumption and Chronic Non-Communicable Diseases-Related Dietary Nutrient Profile in the UK (2008–2014)"*, 2018, US National Library of Medicine National Institutes of Health, viewed 20 January 2022, <www.ncbi.nlm.nih.gov/pmc/articles/PMC5986467/>

4. Imperial College London. "Eating up to ten portions of fruit and vegetables a day may prevent 7.8 million premature deaths worldwide." ScienceDaily, 23 February 2017. <www.sciencedaily.com/releases/2017/02/170223102404.htm>.

5. University of California – San Diego. "Big data from world's largest citizen science microbiome project serves food for thought: How factors such as diet, antibiotics and mental health status can influence the microbial and molecular makeup of your gut." ScienceDaily, 15 May 2018. <www.sciencedaily.com/releases/2018/05/180515092931.htm>

6. NHS, "How to get more fibre into your diet," 2018, NHS, viewed 20 January 2022, <www.nhs.uk/live-well/eat-well/how-to-get-more-fibre-into-your-diet/>

7. Spector, T. D. (2016). The Diet Myth: The real science behind what we eat. London: Weidenfeld & Nicolson.

8. Odegard, I, Sinke, P, Vergeer, R, "TEA of cultivated meat. Future projections for different scenarios," 2021, CE Delft, viewed 20 January 2022, <cedelft.eu/publications/tea-of-cultivated-meat/>

**CHAPTER 9**

1. Murty, C.M, Pittaway, J.K, Ball, M.J, *"Chickpea supplementation in an Australian diet affects food choice, satiety and bowel health,"* 2010, Appetite, viewed 20 January 2022, <pubmed.ncbi.nlm.nih.gov/19945492/>

2. Berners-Lees, M. (2020). How Bad Are Bananas. (rev. ed.), London: Profile Books.

3. Cranfield University, *"100% organic farming could increase greenhouse gas emissions,"* 2019, Cranfield University, viewed 20 January 2022, <www.cranfield.ac.uk/press/news-2019/organic-farming-could-increase-greenhouse-gas-emissions>

**CHAPTER 10**

1. Sharma, S, "Milking the Planet," 2021, Institute for Agriculture and Trade Policy, viewed 20 January 2022, <www.iatp.org/milking-planet>

2. Zhao Y, Martin BR, Weaver CM. "Calcium bioavailability of calcium carbonate fortified soymilk is equivalent to cows' milk in young women". J Nutr. 2005;135(10):2379-2382. doi:10.1093/jn/135.10.2379

3. Trieu K, Bhat S, Dai Z, Leander K, Gigante B, Qian F, et al., "Biomarkers of dairy fat intake, incident cardiovascular disease, and all-cause mortality: A cohort study, systematic review, and meta-analysis," 2021, PLoS Med 18(9): e1003763, viewed 20 January 2022, <doi.org/10.1371/journal.pmed.1003763>

4. Sharma, S, "Milking the Planet," 2021, Institute for Agriculture and Trade Policy, viewed 20 January 2022, <www.iatp.org/milking-planet>

5. Science VS, "Soy, almond, oat milks: are they udder bull?", 2018, Gimlet Media, viewed 20 January 2022, <gimletmedia.com/shows/science-vs/5whmzx>

6. McGiveney, A, "'Like sending bees to war': the deadly truth behind your almond milk obsession," 2020, The Guardian, viewed 20 January 2022, <www.theguardian.com/environment/2020/jan/07/honeybees-deaths-almonds-hives-aoe>

7. Wexler, J, "Is soya sustainable?", 2019, Ethical Consumer, viewed 20 January 2022, <www.ethicalconsumer.org/food-drink/soya-sustainable>

**CHAPTER 11**

1. Hunt, T. (2020). Eating for Pleasure, People and Planet. London: Kyle Books.

2. WRAP, "Wasting food feeds climate change: Food Waste Action Week launches to help tackle climate emergency," 2021, WRAP, viewed 20 January 2022, <wrap.org.uk/media-centre/press-releases/wasting-food-feeds-climate-change-food-waste-action-week-launches-help#>

3. WRAP, 'Food Surplus and Waste in the UK Key Facts,' 2021, WRAP, viewed 28 January 2022, <wrap.org.uk/resources/report/food-surplus-and-waste-uk-key-facts>

4. Food and Agriculture Organization of the United Nations, "The State of Food Security and Nutrition in the World 2021," Food and Agriculture Organization of the United Nations, viewed 20 January 2022, <www.fao.org/state-of-food-security-nutrition>

5. WRAP, "Net Zero: Why resource efficiency holds the answers," 2021, WRAP, viewed 20 January 2022, <wrap.org.uk/sites/default/files/2021-03/WRAP-Net-zero-why-resource-efficiency-holds-the-answers.pdf>

6. WRAP, 'Food Surplus and Waste in the UK Key Facts,' 2021, WRAP, viewed 28 January 2022, <wrap.org.uk/resources/report/food-surplus-and-waste-uk-key-facts>

7. Vision 2020, "Why ban waste food from landfill," 2021, Vision 2020, viewed 20 January 2022, <www.vision2020.info/ban-food-waste/277>

**CHAPTER 12**

1. VT De Vita, TS Lawrence and SA Rosenberg Wolters Kluwer, Cancer: Principles and Practice of Oncology (11th edition), 2019

2. Buchan W. Domestic medicine or a treatise on the prevention and cure of diseases by regimen and simple medicines. London: Strahan W. And Cadell T; 1779. p. 469.276

3. Wright, J. (2020). The Forager's Calendar: A seasonal guide to nature's wild harvest. London: Profile Books.

4. Baldock KCR et al, "A Systems Approach reveals urban pollinator hotspots and conservation opportunities", Nature Ecology and Evolution, 14 January 2019

**CHAPTER 13**

1. Statista, *"Revenue of the beauty & personal care market worldwide from 2012 to 2025"*, 2021, Statista, viewed 20 January 2022, <www.statista.com/forecasts/1244578/beauty-and-personal-care-global-market-value>

2. The Soil Association, "The Organic Market Report 2021," The Soil Association, viewed 20 January 2022, <www.soilassociation.org/certification/market-research-and-data/the-organic-market-report-2021/>

3. Statista, "Advertising spending in the perfumes, cosmetics, and other toilet preparations industry in the United States from 2018 to 2020," 2021, Statista, viewed 20 January 2022, <www.statista.com/statistics/470467/perfumes-cosmetics-and-other-toilet-preparations-industry-ad-spend-usa/>

4. American Chemical Society, *"Sunscreen and cosmetics compound may harm coral by altering fatty acids,"* 9 January 2019, ScienceDaily, viewed 20 January 2022, <www.sciencedaily.com/releases/2019/01/190109110048.htm>

5. Turner, J, "Toxic chemicals in toiletries and beauty products," 2020, Ethical Consumer, viewed 20 January 2022, < www.ethicalconsumer.org/health-beauty/toxic-beauty>

**CHAPTER 14**

1. Woodford, C. (2021). Breathless – why air pollution matters – and how it affects you. Icon Books.

2. Fortune Business Insights, "Household cleaning products market to be worth USD 320.82 billion by 2028; stoked by increasing demand for organic cleaning products," 2021, Globe News Wire, viewed 20 January 2022, <www.globenewswire.com/news-release/2021/06/22/2250982/0/en/Household- Cleaning-Products-Market-to-Worth-USD-320-82-Billion-by-2028-Stoked-by-Increasing- Demand-for-Organic-Cleaning-Products-Says-Fortune-Business-Insights.html>

3. Ethical Consumer, "Toxic chemicals in cleaning products," 2017, Ethical Consumer, viewed 20 January 2022, <www.ethicalconsumer.org/home-garden/toxic-chemicals-cleaning-products>

**CHAPTER 15**

1. Ulrich, R. S., "View through a window may influence recovery from surgery," 1984, Science, volume 224, issue 4647, viewed 29 January 2022, <www.researchgate.net/publication/17043718_View_Through_a_Window_May_Influence_Recovery_from_Surgery>

2. Nalise Hähn, Emmanuel Essah & Tijana Blanusa (2020): Biophilic design and office planting: a case study of effects on perceived health, well-being and performance metrics in the workplace, Intelligent Buildings International, doi: 10.1080/17508975.2020.1732859

3. Woodford, C. (2021). Breathless – why air pollution matters – and how it affects you. Icon Books.

4. Hewitt, C.N., Ashworth, K. & MacKenzie, A.R., "Using green infrastructure to improve urban air quality (GI4AQ)," Ambio 49, 62–73 (2020). <//doi.org/10.1007/s13280-019-01164-3>

5. C. Gubb., T. Blanusa, A. Griffiths, C. Pfrang. "Can houseplants improve indoor air quality by removing $CO_2$ and increasing relative humidity?", 2018.

6. Berners-Lees, M. (2020). How Bad Are Bananas. (rev. ed.), London: Profile Books.

## ABOUT US

Welbeck Balance is dedicated to changing lives.
Our mission is to deliver life-enhancing books to help improve
your wellbeing so that you can live with greater clarity and meaning,
wherever you are on life's journey.

Welbeck Balance is part of the Welbeck Publishing Group –
a globally recognized, independent publisher.
Welbeck are renowned for our innovative ideas, production values
and developing long-lasting content. Our books have been translated
into over 30 languages in more than 60 countries around the world.

If you love books, then join the club and sign up
to our newsletter for exclusive offers, extracts, author interviews
and more information.

To find out more and sign up, visit:

www.welbeckpublishing.com

 welbeckpublish
 welbeckpublish
 welbeckuk

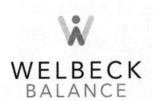

WELBECK
BALANCE